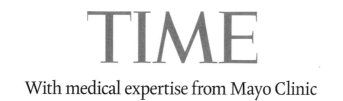

TIME

With medical expertise from Mayo Clinic

Alternative Medicine

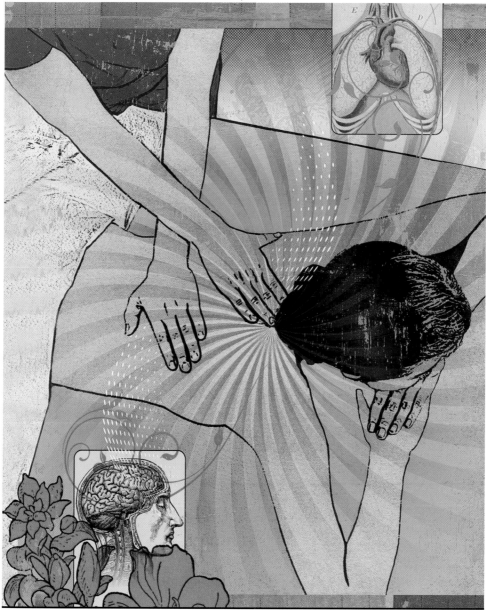

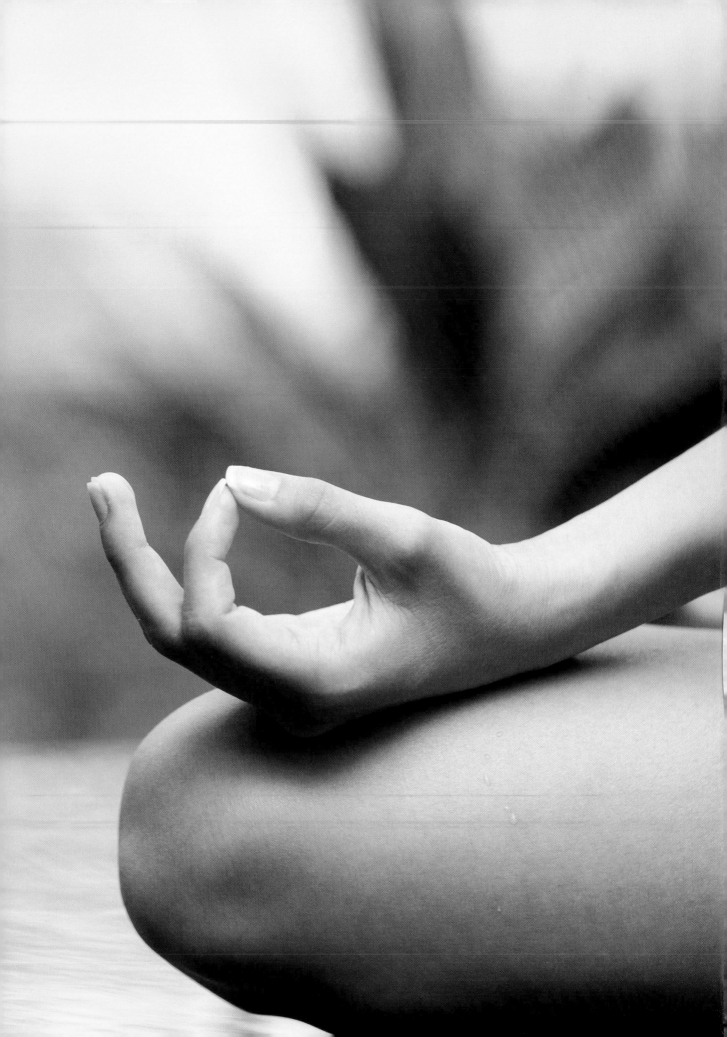

TIME

MANAGING EDITOR Richard Stengel
DESIGN DIRECTOR D.W. Pine
DIRECTOR OF PHOTOGRAPHY Kira Pollack

Alternative Medicine

EDITOR Neil Fine
DESIGNER Arthur Hochstein
PHOTO EDITOR Donna Bender
MEDICAL CONSULTANT Brent Bauer, M.D., Mayo Clinic
WRITERS Lesley Alderman, David Bjerklie, John Cloud, Stacey Colino, Elizabeth Dias, Roseann Foley Henry, Beth Howard, Jeffrey Kluger, M.A. Landau, Lori Oliwenstein, Alice Park, Peg Rosen and Bryan Walsh
REPORTERS Elizabeth L. Bland, Jenisha Watts
COPY EDITORS Jane Sandiford, Shelley Wolson
EDITORIAL PRODUCTION Lionel P. Vargas

TIME HOME ENTERTAINMENT

PUBLISHER Jim Childs
VICE PRESIDENT, BUSINESS DEVELOPMENT AND STRATEGY Steven Sandonato
EXECUTIVE DIRECTOR, MARKETING SERVICES Carol Pittard
EXECUTIVE DIRECTOR, RETAIL AND SPECIAL SALES Tom Mifsud
EXECUTIVE PUBLISHING DIRECTOR Joy Butts
DIRECTOR, BOOKAZINE DEVELOPMENT AND MARKETING Laura Adam
FINANCE DIRECTOR Glenn Buonocore
ASSOCIATE PUBLISHING DIRECTOR Megan Pearlman
ASSISTANT GENERAL COUNSEL Helen Wan
ASSISTANT DIRECTOR SPECIAL SALES Ilene Schreider
BOOK PRODUCTION MANAGER Suzanne Janso
DESIGN AND PREPRESS MANAGER Anne-Michelle Gallero
BRAND MANAGER Michela Wilde
ASSOCIATE PREPRESS MANAGER Alex Voznesenskiy
ASSOCIATE BRAND MANAGER Isata Yansaneh

EDITORIAL DIRECTOR Stephen Koepp
EDITORIAL OPERATIONS DIRECTOR Michael Q. Bullerdick

SPECIAL THANKS TO: Christine Austin, Katherine Barnet, Jeremy Biloon, Stephanie Braga, Susan Chodakiewicz, Rose Cirrincione, Lauren Hall Clark, Jacqueline Fitzgerald, Christine Font, Jenna Goldberg, Hillary Hirsch, David Kahn, Amy Mangus, Robert Marasco, Kimberly Marshall, Amy Migliaccio, Nina Mistry, Stanley Moyse, Dave Rozzelle, Adriana Tierno, Vanessa Wu, TIME Imaging

Copyright © 2012 Time Home Entertainment Inc.
Published by TIME Books, an imprint of Time Home Entertainment Inc.
135 West 50th Street • New York, N.Y. 10020

ISBN 10: 1-61893-017-6
ISBN 13: 978-1-61893-017-0
Library of Congress Number: 2012941936

We welcome your comments and suggestions about TIME Books. Please write to us at:
TIME Books, Attention: Book Editors, P.O. Box 11016, Des Moines, IA 50336-1016

If you would like to order any of our hardcover Collector's Edition books, please call us at 1-800-327-6388, Monday through Friday, 7 a.m. to 8 p.m., or Saturday, 7 a.m. to 6 p.m., Central Time.

FRONT COVER Clockwise, from top left: Kristin Duvall/Getty Images; Rob Daley/Getty Images; Jon Feingersh/Corbis; Ocean/Corbis
BACK COVER Steven Poe/Getty Images

This book is intended as a general reference only, and is not to be used as a substitute for medical advice. We urge you to consult your personal physician regarding any individual medical conditions or specific health issues or questions.

Some of the articles in this book were previously published in substantially the same form in TIME magazine from 2010 through 2012.

Contents

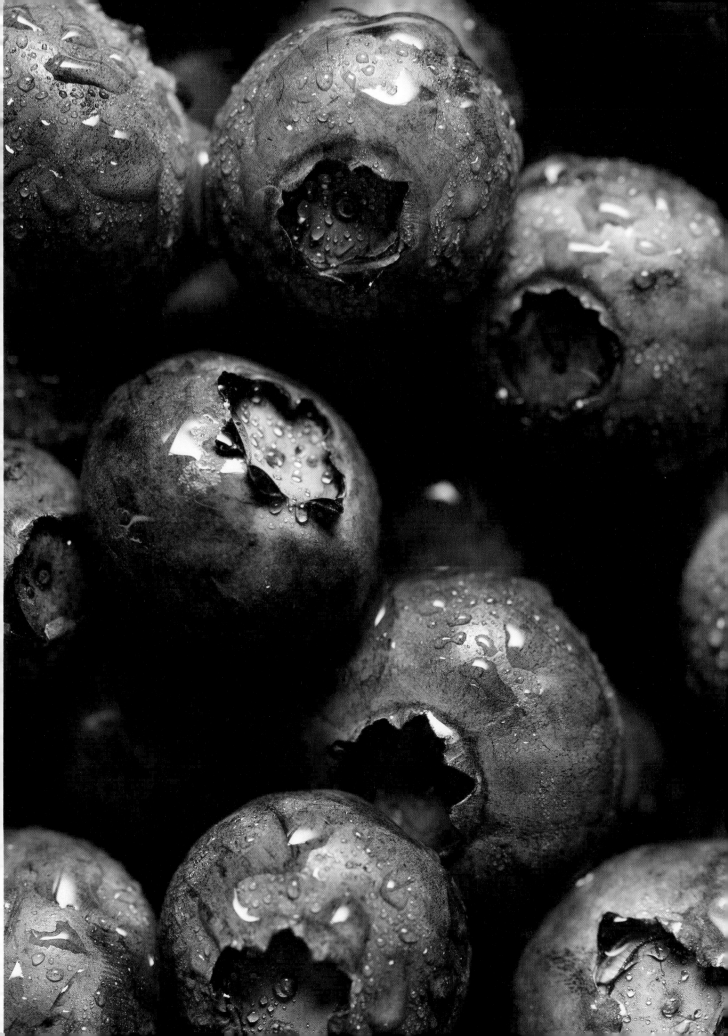

A Healthy New Approach To What Ails You

By Brent Bauer, M.D.

WAS THERE EVER A NARROWER, MORE LIMITING TERM THAN "alternative"—an idea defined by that which it is not? From the word alone, you have no idea what you're getting—only what's being left out. That has long been a challenge for what is commonly called alternative medicine. The medicine most of us are familiar with involves pills and shots, surgery and x-rays, and all the other tested, peer-reviewed stuff that on the whole does a pretty good job of making us well. So alternative medicine is what? Untested nonsense that leaves us no better than before?

Assuredly not. For one thing, the treatments that stand outside of what is still the mainstream —yoga, meditation, herbs, acupuncture, massage, and more—have a long and robust history. For another—let's be honest—doesn't Western medicine have some room for improvement?

The explosion in technological advances over the past decades has undeniably transformed medical science. But even as old scourges (think polio) are driven to near extinction and existing plagues (think cancer and AIDS) increasingly yield to better treatments, other afflictions, like obesity and diabetes, rise up to create new health crises. And as we rely more and more on pharmaceutical solutions to our ills, some drugs, like antibiotics, have grown less effective, while others lead to unwanted side effects. At the same time, many patients find the practice of medicine is growing colder, less personal, and that has spurred them to take more control of their own care by exploring options a doctor may not be mentioning in those eight-minute office visits.

This upsurge in self-treatment can be a good thing. Someone receiving narcotics for a pain problem might do well with a little hypnosis on the side. Someone taking antihistamines for allergies might also be irrigating with a Neti pot. Someone recovering from major surgery might also tap music therapy to heal. In the 1990s this mix-and-match method gave birth to a new term in the health-care field: "complementary and alternative medicine," or CAM. Not only was it more inclusive than "alternative medicine," but it also acknowledged what was really happening in doctor's offices, emergency rooms, and patients' homes. CAM treatments weren't replacing mainstream medicine, they were supplementing it.

In 1991 the National Center for Complementary and Alternative Medicine (NCCAM) was launched, under the aegis of the National Institutes of Health, with a mission "to define, through rigorous scientific investigation, the usefulness and safety of complementary- and alternative-medicine interventions and their roles in improving health and health care." NCCAM set about sponsoring research—and conducting its own—to confirm or refute the effectiveness of these sporadically studied therapies. Before long, results began pouring in—and the news they brought was encouraging.

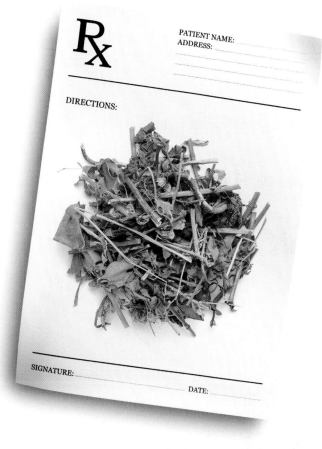

The state of the art: Doctors now complement traditional medicine with alternative disciplines such as Chinese herbs (above).

As we describe in TIME's *Alternative Medicine*, for which Mayo Clinic served as the main provider of medical expertise, an ever-growing body of peer-reviewed studies is validating a host of CAM protocols. That's good, but it can lull the uninitiated into a false sense of security. Herbs and other complementary remedies, for example, are still not regulated in the same way that pharmaceuticals are; they're available to anyone, bolstered by unsubstantiated claims from an enthusiast or huckster with access to a cable show or Internet site. One low point occurred in 2000 when it was reported that two recovering heart-transplant patients who used St. John's wort (an effective herbal treatment for mild to moderate depression) experienced transplant rejection. It turned out that St. John's wort is a powerful inducer of liver enzymes that can counter the effect of anti-rejection medications. Other natural medications have caused patients to experience bleeding, seizures, and arrhythmias.

Such episodes underscore the need for CAM treatments to be examined closely and brought more fully into the fold of the existing health-care system. It's an idea that has already spawned yet another term—"integrative" medicine—which better captures the hybrid nature of the new thinking. And what it describes is nothing less than a sea change.

I've served as the director of Mayo Clinic's Integrative Medicine Program since 2001. During that time my colleagues and I have conducted more than 100 studies on integrative techniques that have increasingly persuaded us that this third way works—and works well. Just last year more than 18,000 patients at Mayo received acupuncture, massage, or meditation training. Mayo isn't the only visionary hospital in the U.S. with a thriving integrative-medicine program. We just like to think we're the best. But whatever the merits of any particular program, the merits of the integrative idea are real and growing. No book can explore every corner of the field, but this one will shine a helpful light across the current landscape, showing you new ways to get well now—and stay that way.

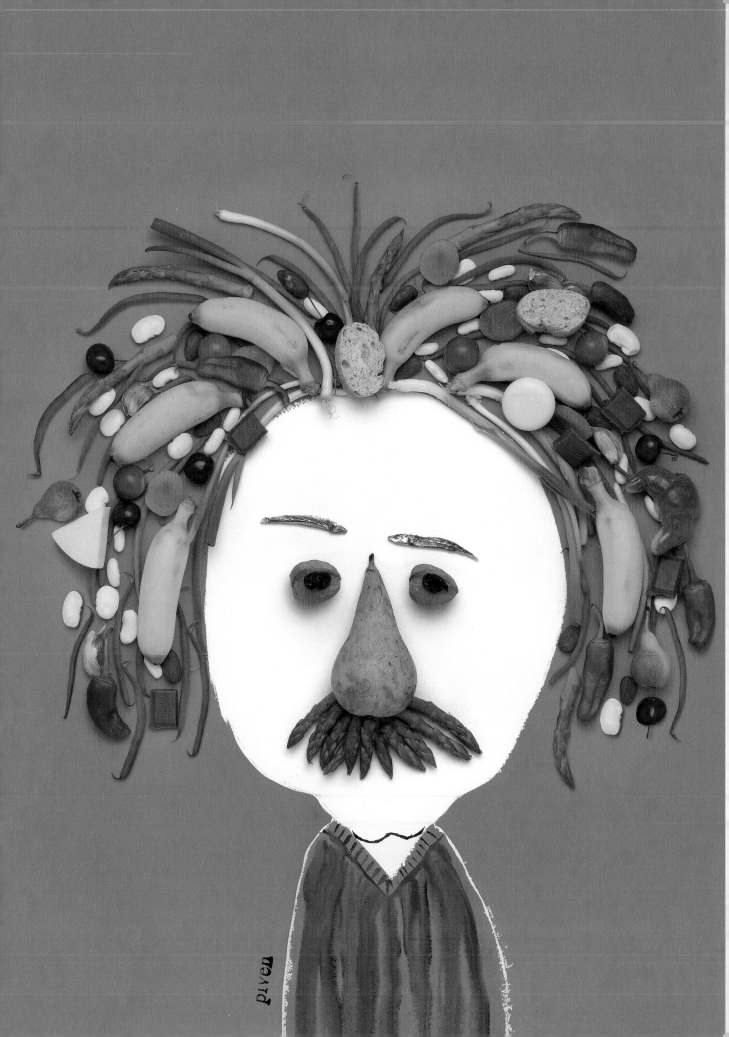

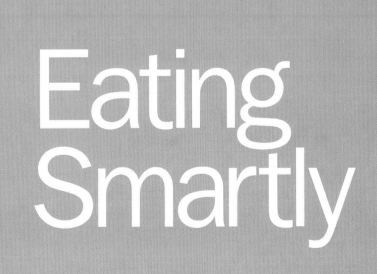

Eating Smartly

Your Friendly Microbes

Turns out your body is host to a whole world of organisms. How to make probiotics work for you.
By Alice Park

SCIENCE HAS LEFT FEW FRONTIERS UNCHARTED IN THE HUMAN body. CT and PET scans allow us to peer through flesh into bones and organs. Genetic tests help us decipher the molecular instructions that guide cell growth. We can even watch the brain at work with MRIs that record neurons as they fire in the perfected choreography of cognition. And yet one vast universe remains largely unexplored, a world where interlopers outnumber homegrown cells by a factor of 10, and the DNA of which is composed of a whopping 8 million genes (humans, in comparison, have a paltry 23,000). It's the microbial kingdom, an invisible ecosystem that can have profound effects on our health, influencing everything from our risk of cancer and obesity to immune disorders, asthma, colds, flu, and maybe even autism.

We tend to think of this unseen underworld as an army of disease-

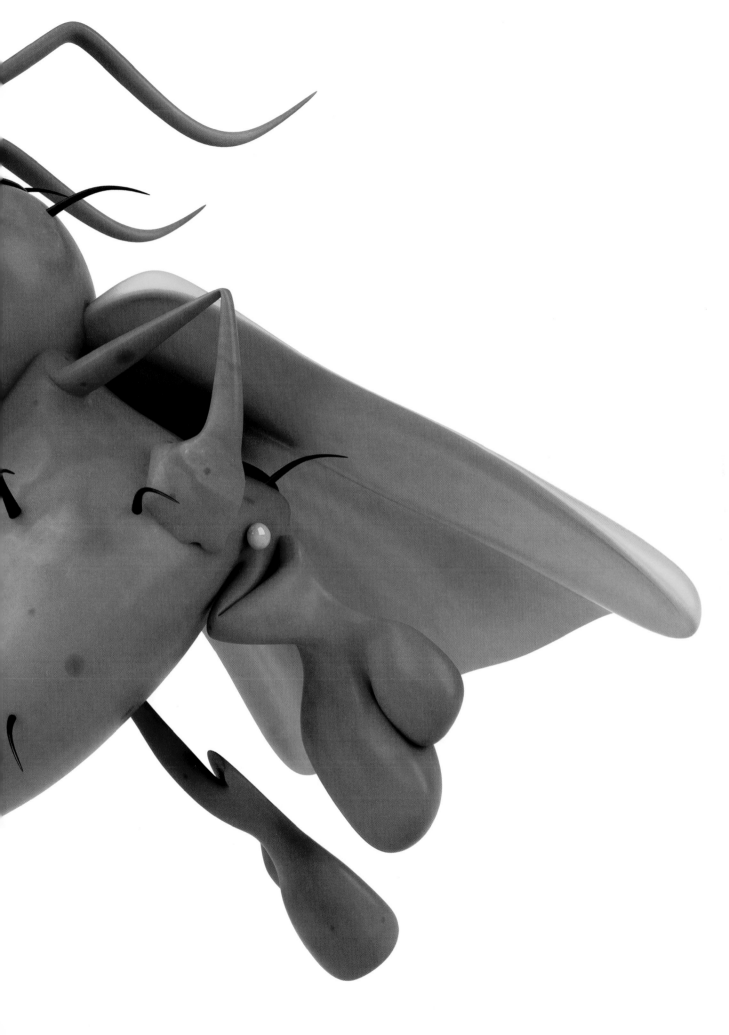

A Helping Of Probiotics

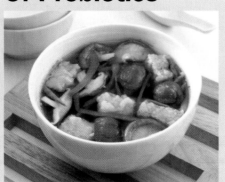

Miso, the traditional Japanese soy seasoning, is a good source of probiotics

Although the study of probiotics continues, early indications are that most people tolerate them well (children, the elderly, and those with compromised immune systems may want to stay away until we know more). So here are some ways to add a little probiotic flavor to your everyday diet.

- Mix plain yogurt or kefir (a fermented milk drink) with fruit and a little sweetener for a snack or dessert or as a base for smoothies and ice cream.

- Use miso, a soy-based seasoning, in soups, marinades, and salad dressings. Another soy product, tempeh, can sub for meat in sandwiches, spaghetti, or chili.

- Top a sandwich or accompany an entrée with sauerkraut.

- Feel free to treat yourself to a bar of good-quality dark chocolate or a glass of wine—but only once in a while.

- Thirsty? Search out probiotic soy beverages and fruit drinks in your local supermarket.

- Probiotic supplements, in capsule and powder form, are available. But use them only as directed and after consulting a caregiver.

- Antibiotics may go after your body's good bacteria as well, so when your doctor prescribes them, ask about taking a probiotic supplement too. But be sure to take the medications at least two hours apart.

- Similarly, some foods may promote the growth of your local flora. These prebiotics include wheat, barley, oats, chicory root, artichoke, banana, garlic, onion, and honey.

By Charla Schultz, Registered Dietitian, Mayo Clinic Department of Endocrinology

carrying invaders—bacteria, viruses, and other pathogens that have us sniffling in bed or moaning in the emergency room. The fact is, though, evildoing microbes are the exception. The vast majority of bugs that live in, on, and around us are good neighbors—allies, actually—performing functions essential to good health. "Tens of thousands of species of microorganisms live with us," says Lita Proctor, coordinator of the Human Microbiome Project at the National Institutes of Health (NIH). "They belong there, they're good for us, and they support health and well-being."

Consider the microbes that reside in the gut, by far the human body's largest community of tiny tenants. Most are bacteria with odd-sounding names like Firmicutes and Bacteroidetes, but they perform the vital function of producing enzymes that break down plant fibers. Without them, we wouldn't be able to absorb the nutrients and vitamins found in leafy vegetables and legumes. Other bacteria ferment digested food in our intestines, helping transform what we eat into the energy our cells need.

The goal of so much of the medicine we take and therapies we undergo is to rid the body of microbes. But now that we are beginning to realize the benefits of these organisms, scientists are developing treatments that do just the opposite: seed the body with them. This blossoming field, known as probiotics, shares its name with the class of "good" bacteria it uses, and its potential as a wellness tool is virtually limitless.

Our relationship with beneficial microbes goes back a long way, to our very first moments in the world. The womb is a sterile environment; delivery is a newborn's first confrontation with germs. Over the course of a pregnancy, the makeup of the bacteria in the vagina—the vaginal microbiome—changes, and by the end of nine months it's a well-represented community of bugs that an infant is likely to encounter in the outside world. This initial inoculation primes a baby's immune system to identify potentially troublesome pathogens and mount appropriate immune responses against them.

The journey through the birth canal is an important one. Intriguing preliminary evidence

Eat yogurt in sufficient amounts, and its active cultures may help promote digestive health.

suggests that the makeup of the vaginal microbiome can influence a child's later health, possibly causing, for instance, the development of asthma and allergies. Similarly, scientists hope to tease out microbial "profiles" that characterize babies who might be susceptible to certain illnesses; some research suggests that gut microbes adjust to what we eat and react to the air we breathe and illnesses we encounter.

Figuring out how these microbial populations respond to stimuli will open whole new treatment paths, and maybe even help us avoid sickness in the first place. In 2007, the NIH invested $153 million in the Human Microbiome Project. Modeled after the Human Genome Project, which sequenced the body's genes, the current undertaking will map all the microbes that live in our gut, nose, mouth, and reproductive tracts. So far, 5,000 samples from 200 people have been analyzed.

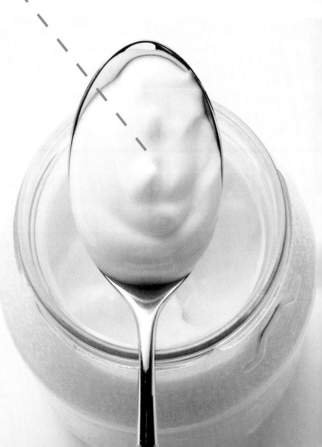

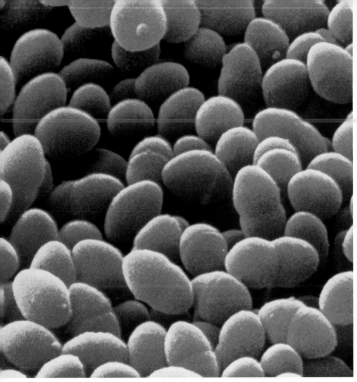

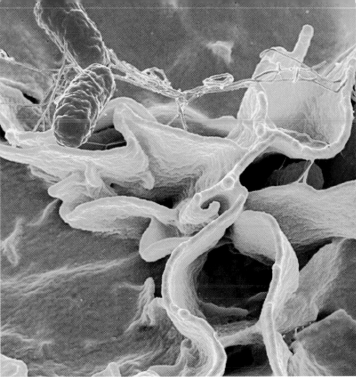

ENTEROCOCCI
Found in the vaginal and intestinal regions of 40% to 80% of individuals, some strains of this bacterium cause infection, but many others make our immune system more efficient.

SALMONELLA
Unlike E. coli, salmonella fully deserves its bad reputation. A lot of what we call food poisoning comes from strains that are found mostly in raw eggs and chicken but can turn up almost anywhere. In the worst cases, salmonella poisoning kills.

Good Germs, Bad Germs
Some bugs deserve their bad reputations, while others do not. Our bodies have both kinds in abundance.

The researchers hope to create a database of microbes that will help link particular communities to either disease or improved health. "This is a vast territory we've never studied," says George Weinstock, associate director of the Genome Institute at Washington University in St. Louis.

Why has so much remained out of reach until now? For starters, many of the bacteria are difficult, if not impossible, to grow outside the inviting confines of the human body. That has made it challenging for microbiologists to get an accurate tally of what resides within us, much less figure out what the organisms do. But advances in DNA sequencing now allow researchers to bypass culturing altogether. Essentially, they use genetics to take bacterial attendance, filtering out recognizable human genes from a sample, then logging the remaining DNA. The latest investigations have uncovered some tantalizing clues about the dramatic effects this microworld can have on our health. Scientists have learned, for example, that obese people and people of normal weight harbor different bacteria in their intes-

tines, and that the composition of bacterial communities changes depending on what you eat. People who favor high-fat, low-fiber diets tend to house more Bacteroidetes bugs, while those who eat less animal fat show higher concentrations of Prevotella microbes. From a therapeutic perspective, it would be important to know if this relationship works the other way too; that is, can different types of gut flora influence or even change eating habits?

What does seem to be true is that tweaking a person's microbial profile can improve his health. Studies hint that probiotics, in particular lactic acid bacteria and bifidobacteria, can thwart cold and flu viruses, resulting in 12% fewer respiratory infections among children and adults given them, compared with a control group. More encouraging, probiotics may help cold and flu sufferers reduce their antibiotic dosage—a huge plus given the growing problem of antibiotic-resistant bugs.

In another recent treatment advance, patients with C. difficile infections, which can cause per-

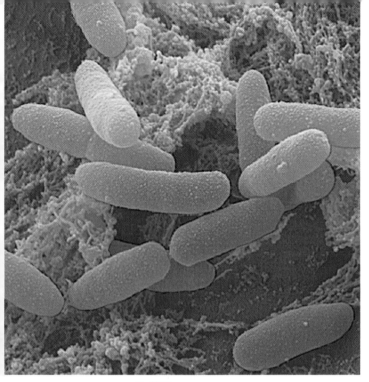

E. COLI
This is a much-maligned bacterium, and for good reason: It can cause deadly disease. But that's not the whole story. Some strains, naturally occurring in our abdominal tract, aid digestion and keep bad microbes at bay.

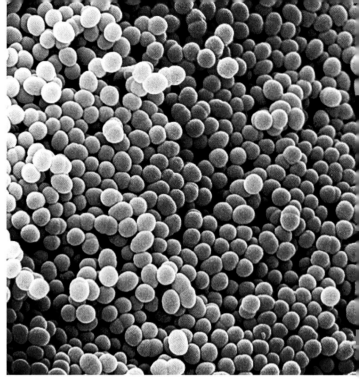

STAPHYLOCOCCUS AUREUS
Although most of us carry the bacteria on our skin, it can turn deadly if it enters the body, particularly if a person has compromised immunity.

sistent diarrhea, abdominal cramping, and fever, have been administered fecal transplants. Yes, that is just what it sounds like: infusions of feces from an uninfected, usually related, donor. While the procedure may seem unpleasant—best to think of it as a kind of enema—it's hard to argue with the nearly 80% cure rate.

Similarly, doctors at some cancer centers advise patients to bank stool samples—essentially, a concentrated form of their microbiome—before chemotherapy, just as they might store blood for transfusions, to replenish what the toxic treatment wipes out. Early studies show that patients who do this rebound quicker from their chemo course than those who don't.

Then again, doctors don't expect fecal transplants to become as common as flu shots. "I think that in the not-too-distant future we will be able to have probiotics or dietary supplements to support beneficial microbes," says Proctor. Some of those may be composed entirely of strains of probiotics, while others, known as synbiotics, may be combinations of probiotics and prebiotics. Prebiotics aren't microbes at all, but rather indigestible parts of the foods we eat (say, the fiber in whole grains) that nourish the good bacteria.

Some consumer-ready probiotics may already exist in our grocer's dairy case. The makers of Activia yogurt say their product eases digestive disorders by repopulating the stomach with healthful bacterial colonies. Then again, they may have gotten a little ahead of themselves, having landed in court as defendants in a class action suit that alleged false and misleading advertising claims.

That doesn't mean those claims won't eventually be proved true, though. Once we fully understand how microbes morph in response to what we do and what we eat, not to mention environmental factors, we will be able to manipulate them to our benefit. Further, many of these bacteria interact with each other to produce enzymes, digest food, and fight inflammation, intimately connecting them to the body's metabolic processes. Playing on that field—tweaking the pathways by which compounds and chemicals pass back and forth—will lead to the most significant advances.

Imagine being able to overcome obesity simply by adjusting the makeup of the gut's ecosystem. Or saving patients from a fatal infection by giving them some microbes to ingest? That's the promise of the human microbiome, the hidden world that isn't likely to remain out of sight for long.

The Dirty Little Secret of Dietary Cleanses

From fasts to flushes, many of us will do whatever it takes to cleanse our body of toxins. But what if we don't have to do anything at all? By Peg Rosen

"I JUST FINISHED A DETOX, AND I FEEL AMAZING."

Brent Bauer, director of the Mayo Clinic Integrative Medicine Program in Rochester, Minn., hears some version of this sentiment pretty frequently these days. He believes what his patients are telling him. He even understands the motivation behind their "cleanses," the practice of subsisting for days on green shakes, highly restrictive diets, or even plain water to rid the body of impurities. "We put a lot into our bodies that isn't healthy," Bauer says. Indeed, even for people who are paying attention, a scary cocktail of contaminants makes its way into our system through what we eat and what we breathe. A recent report by the Centers for Disease Control and Prevention found that a multitude of potentially harmful substances—including fire retardants, hydrocarbons, and epoxy resins—were present in the blood or urine of most of its study subjects.

"It's tempting to think you can do something to clear out what's built up in your

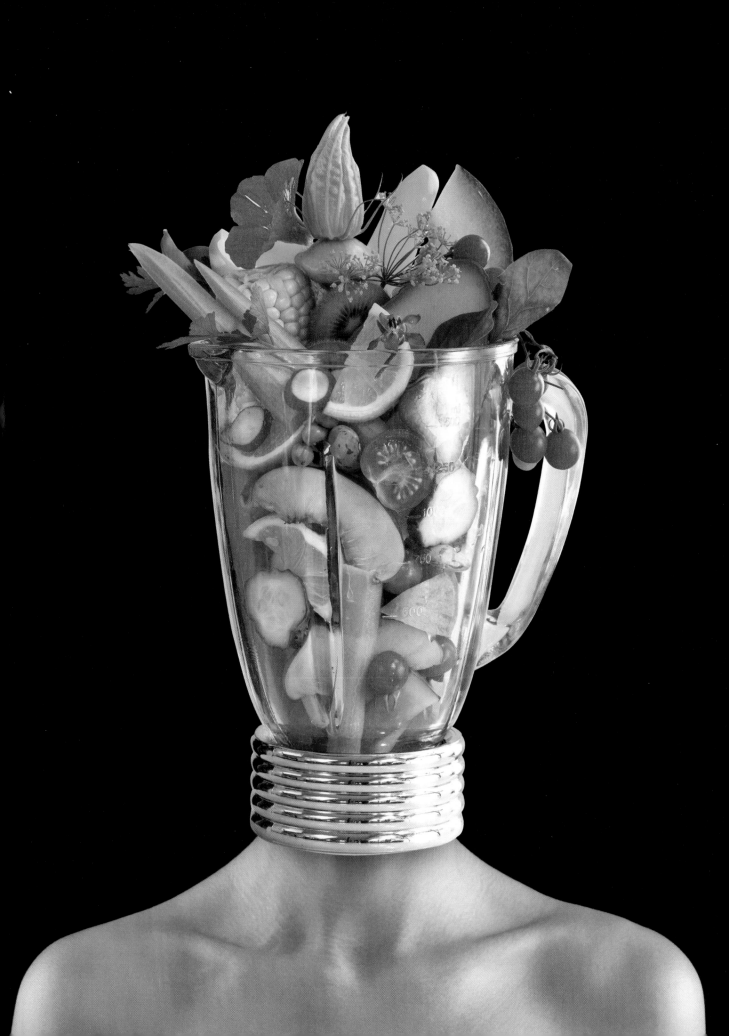

body," Bauer says. "People spend a lot of money on products or regimens that supposedly do this." As far as he is concerned, there's just one catch: "I've yet to have a single patient who can provide any evidence that a 'detox' actually cleared toxins from their system or, for that matter, tell me exactly what toxins they were worried about in the first place."

There is no question that toxins (chemicals or microorganisms from within or without the body) can make us ill or otherwise do us harm. But there is little research to support the notion that any attempt to "detox" from them—unless, they are, say, addictive substances like drugs or alcohol—is effective. Or even necessary.

The fact is, the human body does a decent job of scrubbing itself clean all on its own. Our liver, kidneys, lungs, and skin exist in large part to filter out impurities, eliminating them in sweat, urine, breath, and feces. Bacteria in the colon neutralize food waste, and that organ's mucous lining prevents potentially harmful organisms and waste products from seeping back into our system. And while some toxins are absorbed by fat cells—where they can take up permanent residence—there's little evidence to suggest that fasting, sweating, drinking special potions, or flushing will cast them out.

"Cleansing," though, is no here-today fad. Ancient Egyptians purged their colons at specific times during the lunar cycle. Later, the Greeks believed that eating allowed "demonic forces" to enter the body and embraced fasting as an antidote. In 1894, E.H. Dewey wrote in *The True Science of Living* that "every disease that afflicts mankind [develops from] more or less habitual eating in excess of the supply of gastric juice." And celebrated early-20th-century muckraker Upton Sinclair sparked an unprecedented reader response with two articles he wrote for *Cosmopolitan* magazine in praise of therapeutic fasting. He said he was compelled to compile his stories in a book, *The Fasting Cure*, to avoid having to answer "half a dozen 'fasting letters' every day for the rest of my life."

Today therapeutic cleansing is once again in the limelight, with a little extra sparkle, thanks to a flock of A-list advocates. Both Salma Hayek and Gwyneth Paltrow are passionate juice cleansers; Hayek even peddles her own signature concoctions. Then-marrieds Demi Moore and Ashton Kutcher dabbled in cleanses. Michelle Obama has confessed to a fondness for fruit-and-veggie cleanses. And Jennifer Aniston, Halle Berry, and Britney Spears are all reported fans of colonics. We want to be like them and look like them. And if that means shelling out big bucks, denying ourselves solid food, or lying naked on a table as gallons of water are pumped into our colons, we're willing to cleanse like them!

Is less more?

All hype aside, the idea that dramatically restricting what goes into the body, at least for a limited time, may be beneficial isn't totally unreasonable. "There is a decent amount of research on fasting. Threads of evidence suggest there may be some benefits," says Mary Beth Augustine, senior integrative nutritionist at the Continuum Center for Health and Healing at Beth Israel Medical Center in New York City. Animal studies have shown that intermittent fasting slows brain aging and reduces cancer risk. And research presented at a 2011 meeting of the American College of Cardiology suggested that periodic fasting may also trigger changes in metabolism that lower the risk of coronary heart disease and diabetes.

But that study, too, comes with a significant qualification. "We're talking about a cumulative effect here," says Benjamin Horne, lead author of the study and director of cardiovascular and genetic epidemiology at the Intermountain Heart Institute in Salt Lake City. "Fasting a couple of times isn't going to do the same thing. The promises that some juice fasts and fasting books make are over the top and unrealistic."

What are those promises exactly? Well, purveyors of traditional juice fasts—regimens that involve drinking vegetable and fruit juices exclusively or with limited amounts of solid food—claim weight loss, relief from bloating, the elimination of unspecified toxins, a general boost to the immune system, and in some cases a reduced

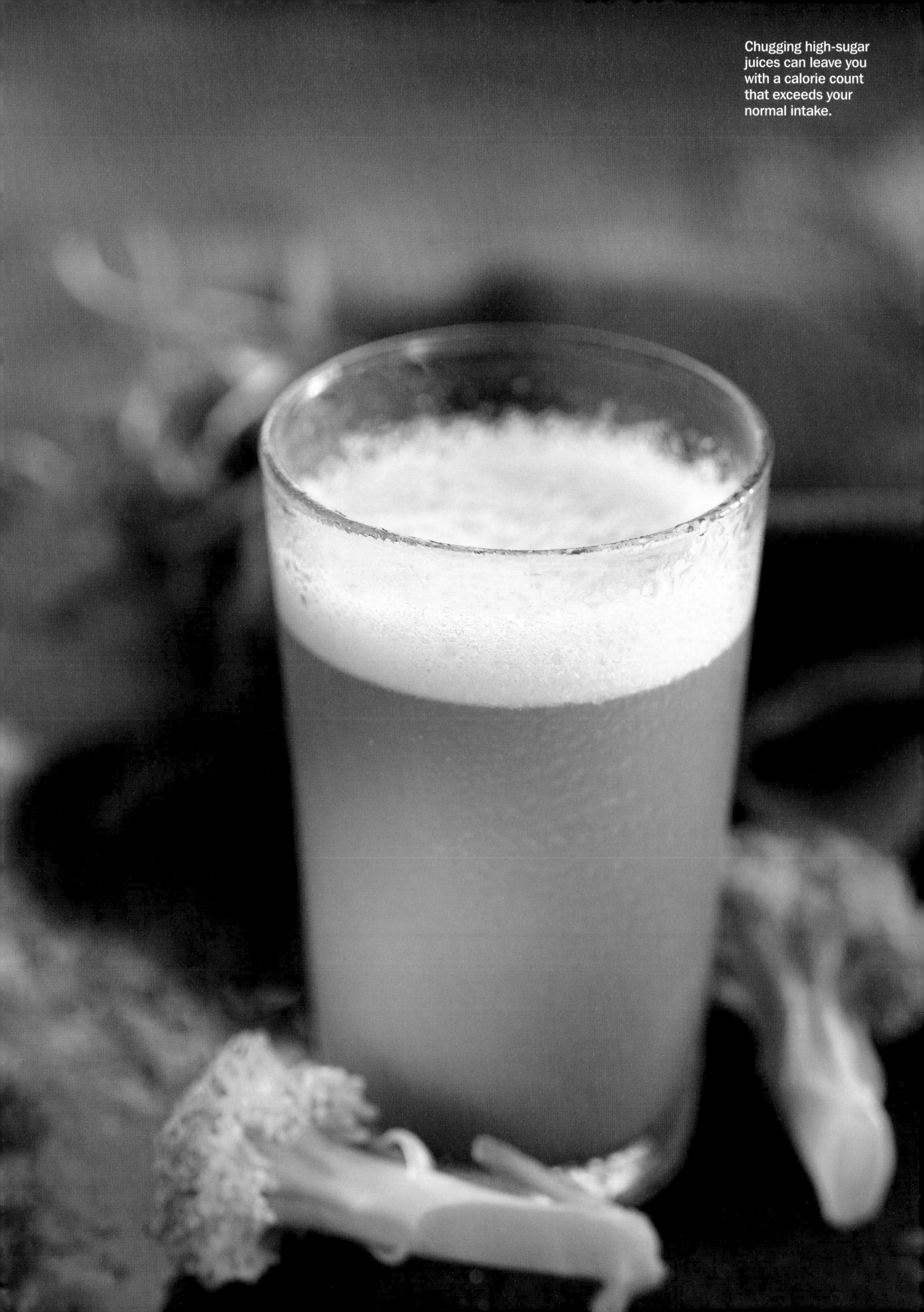

Chugging high-sugar juices can leave you with a calorie count that exceeds your normal intake.

risk of cancer and other diseases. One modified juice fast, the Master Cleanse (also known as the lemonade diet because it features a concoction of lemon juice, maple syrup, cayenne pepper, and water) purports to also flush undigested food and built-up waste from the body. According to one testimonial, the waste included items swallowed as a child.

Food-based detox diets, a regimented intake of a limited variety of edibles—particular fruits and vegetables, nuts, whole grains, maybe a little fish, and sometimes supplemented with digestive enzymes and laxatives—allegedly expunge targeted disease-causing bacteria (like Candida), or cleanse particular organs (like the liver) of stored impurities. The draw of colonics, also known as colonic irrigation or colonic hydrotherapy, may be more visceral. The goal of this process, in which as much as 15 gallons of fluid are flushed through the colon by means of a tube inserted in the rectum, is to remove fecal matter that has built up in the digestive tract. Backers of this treatment buy into the theory of "autointoxication," which holds that fecal toxins leach back into the body, causing a range of maladies from fatigue to allergies.

Liver flushes, too, profess to offer tangible results. These oral home remedies or purchased formulas, usually containing some combination of oil and acid, promise to rid the body of fat-soluble toxins, parasites, and other impurities such as gallstones. After a couple of days, the flusher sees green gelatinous "stones" in the stool—theoretically, evidence of excreted toxins. Some testimonials cite as many as 200 evacuated stones.

It all sounds so impressive. If only more than the barest minimum of it were true. Sure, other-wise healthy individuals may feel less bloated or lose weight on many of these routines. But think about it: These fasts and diets by definition restrict caloric intake and specifically exclude processed foods, caffeine, alcohol, fatty animal protein, and excess sodium. What health professional would argue with that regimen? If you feel good on a juice fast, it's probably because of what you are *not* consuming.

Then again, chugging so many high-sugar juices can quickly leave you with a calorie count that exceeds your normal nonfasting one. And, more broadly, there is simply no proof that the regimens cleanse organs, reduce fat, or expel toxins. Autointoxication, by the way, was debunked by the American Medical Association—in 1919. And the stones that are produced during those liver flushes? Nothing more than the congealed byproduct of the flush's ingredients. In any case, the human body just doesn't host that much built-up waste—as anybody who has ever peered into a colonoscope will confirm.

On the plus side, few of the therapies are especially risky for healthy individuals—with the exception of colon therapy. An improperly administered colonic may result in a host of complications, ranging from bowel perforation and infection to reduced kidney function, electrolyte abnormalities, and possibly even heart and kidney failure. Vomiting, dehydration, and the obliteration of helpful bacteria that keep the bowel environment in healthy balance have also been reported.

Liver flushes can lead to explosive diarrhea—not to mention the revulsion that comes from inspecting one's own feces for gelatinous green lumps. In rare instances, a flush may cause cramping that dislodges a gallstone that then dangerously becomes stuck in a bile duct. Really,

Before You Cleanse …

The benefit of detoxing therapies is far from certain, and the last thing you want to do is cause yourself harm by trying one. So be sure to take these precautions.

- Check with your conventional medical provider before you undertake detoxing, especially if you are on medications or have health problems.

- If you choose to do a colon cleanse, make sure your practitioner uses a set of disposable equipment that hasn't been used previously.

- Research the list of any herbal ingredients and the amounts called for in any colon-cleansing product you are thinking about using—some of them can cause side effects.

- Drink lots of fluids while undergoing a cleanse to prevent dehydration.

— *Michael F. Picco, M.D., Mayo Clinic*

Famous Flushers A yen to cleanse has caught on with celebrities. But beware—their testimonials are by no means irrefutable.

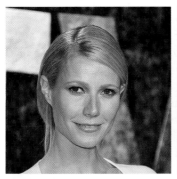

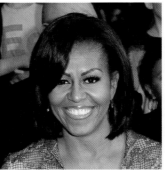

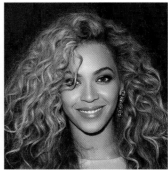

Gwyneth Paltrow claims annual detoxes help keep her slim.

An occasional two-day fruit-and-veggie plan suits Michelle Obama.

Beyoncé dropped 20 pounds for a movie role on the lemonade diet.

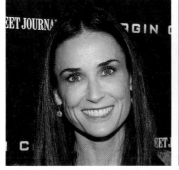

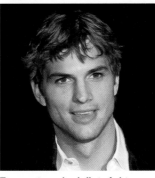

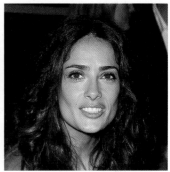

Demi Moore once tried a 10-day liquid fast to flush out toxins.

To counter a bad diet, Ashton Kutcher did a Master Cleanse.

For Salma Hayek, juice cleanses are a motivator to eat healthier.

though, the biggest downside of these flushes, specifically when they are used to eradicate gallstones, is that they delay individuals from seeking more conventional treatment.

But those are worst-case scenarios of more extreme therapies. For people in generally good health who aren't pregnant, breastfeeding, or severely underweight, juice fasts of a few days, or even weeklong restricted cleanse diets, won't hurt. In fact, they might even do some good beyond short-term weight loss (which, in any case, results mostly from loss of water and sodium, not fat).

Many cleansers experience post-treatment exhilaration. It might be nothing more than a placebo effect, but that's okay; you can ride that feeling and jump-start more permanent dietary and lifestyle changes. "It's one reason why—even if it's not my choice as a first-line treatment—I

support my patients who want to try it," says Augustine. Because in the end, of course, it's long-term, consistently maintained dietary changes that make us healthier. Anyone in the cleansing game for a quick fix, to shed pounds or counteract recent bouts of overindulgence, is wasting his time. And that's mostly because the majority of cleansers revert to old habits after treatment, often with a vengeance. Whatever pounds were lost are gained right back. Worse, that can trigger a vicious cycle of yo-yo dieting in an effort to hold one's ground.

"My clients often come in telling me they want to do a cleanse to get back on track," says Andrea Giancoli, a spokeswoman for the Academy of Nutrition and Dietetics. "But why not just do something that gets you on track and allows you to stay there? If you really want to do a cleanse, cleanse your fridge and your pantry."

Nutrition In a Pill

I took 3,000 supplements over five months.
Here's what happened. *By John Cloud*

THE FIRST QUESTION ISN'T WHY, BUT WHY NOT? VITAMINS, PROBIOTICS, omega-3 capsules, antioxidant pills: They can't hurt, right? Around the corner of each advancing birthday lurks a possible affliction—arthritis, cancer, Alzheimer's—and a giant industry has emerged to try to prevent them all. Americans spend something like $28 billion a year on dietary supplements, more than twice what we spent in 1995 and more than $5 billion more than what we pay each year for gym memberships. But do supplements actually work? Dietary supplements occupy the broad, poorly regulated space between two more-defined kinds of consumables: foods and drugs. Because they can and sometimes do provide both nutrition without eating and wellness without medicine, supplements have acquired a new name in recent years: nutraceuticals. When I turned 40 not long ago, I decided to subject myself to a nutraceutical regimen. For five months I took 22 pills a day. There were also protein bars, powder drinks, and enough psyllium fiber to regulate an elephant—but before

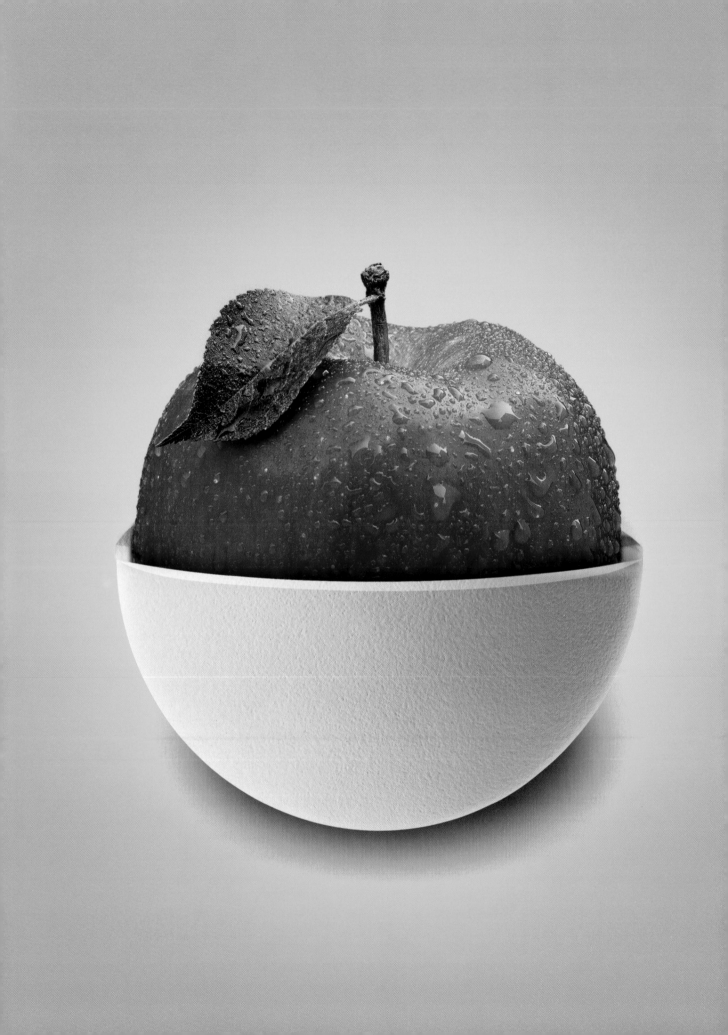

I took anything, I got a blood test. A lab measured the baseline levels of calcium, protein, sodium, cholesterol, and other substances in my blood. After five months and more than 3,000 pills, I had another blood test to see what, if anything, had changed.

I didn't randomly pick the pills I took. A highly lucrative trend in the nutraceutical business is a personalized approach. You provide the supplement company with details of your eating habits and medical history, and it sells you a customized suite of products. (No supplement company I found actually looks at blood results in advance.) If you don't eat much fish, you'll get an omega-3 pill. If you have trouble sleeping, melatonin is on the way.

Whether nutraceuticals improve health—and how—is a matter of enormous scientific inquiry. New studies emerge regularly. Take one typical week in 2010: the *Journal of Clinical Oncology* published the results of a Stanford study showing that a tablet with calcium and vitamin D may lower the chances of getting skin cancer. The same day, the Public Library of Science (PLOS) reported that a compound called fisetin, which is found in strawberries, reduces the severity of complications from diabetes. Three days later a team of 18 researchers from France and the U.S. announced that a daily dose of resveratrol—a substance found in grapes that winemakers love to tout—may help prevent loss of bone mineral density.

And yet all three studies turned out to have shortcomings common in nutraceutical research. The Stanford paper was based on just 176 women, chosen because they had a history of a specific type of skin cancer. The PLOS study, as well as the France-U.S. one, looked only at rodents. When I met with Dr. Glenn Braunstein, chairman of the department of medicine at Cedars-Sinai Medical Center in Los Angeles and an expert on nutraceuticals, he was frank about the state of the research. Overall, he said, "the data is lousy." Many nutraceutical studies have tiny sample sizes and lack placebo controls. Braunstein added that because some supplements have 10 or more ingredients, it's difficult to determine which ingredient is doing what.

So I was surprised when Braunstein revealed that he takes a nutraceutical product, a tablet containing 2,000 international units of vitamin D. What about all that stuff about poor sample sizes and placebo controls? He said a growing body of high-quality literature is showing that even people who live in sunny climates can have low vitamin-D levels. (When exposed to sun, the body naturally produces vitamin D.) He also said that even though he is an avid runner, he discovered not long ago that his blood contained 26 nanograms per milliliter (ng/ml) of vitamin D, below the 30 ng/ml level that many doctors see as a healthy baseline. After he started taking the supplement, his score shot into the high 30s. My vitamin-D measure also skyrocketed when I took nutraceuticals: I went from 28 ng/ml in January to 49 ng/ml in June.

So it turns out that some nutraceuticals do work, at least enough for a skeptical medical department chairman to take a daily just-in-case dose. Braunstein said there's debate in the medical community over whether 30 ng/ml is really the right benchmark for vitamin D, but all the questions led me back to the original one. Why not take supplements just to be safe? Admittedly, that's more a question of faith than of science, a question that recalls a classic discussion about religion: If you go to services every week, but it turns out there's no God, no harm done. But if you choose a reckless path, you burn for eternity. So just swallow the pill, right?

Health by the carton

The boxes arrived just before my first blood test. The cardboard was crisp, and the tape perfectly cornered. But it was like a disappointing Christmas. Each box contained pills and powders and fake-food bars. There were so many that I had to start stacking them under the bed.

A few weeks earlier I had completed an online evaluation for Usana Health Sciences, a Salt Lake City–based supplement maker that has provided nutraceuticals for the U.S. Olympic Ski Team, the Women's Tennis Association, and boxer Manny Pacquiao. The company posted $582 million in

The writer took these eight pills every morning, and 14 more throughout the rest of the day.

PROFLAVINOL C 200
Mix of grape seed extract
and vitamin C claims to
offer heart health.

PROCOSA II
A blend of vitamins
and minerals meant to
support joint fitness.

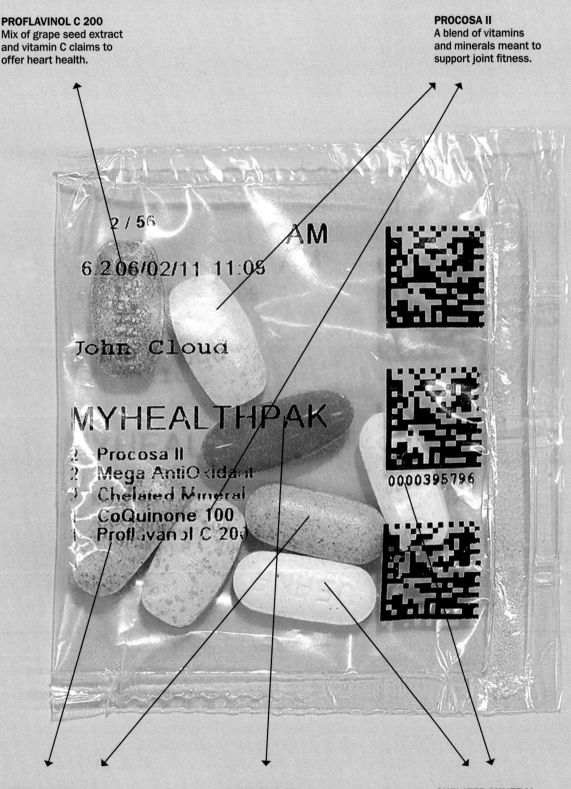

MEGA ANTIOXIDANT
Provides a wide range of
antioxidants, including
vitamins C and E.

COQUINONE 100
An enzyme that fuels
the production of energy
in heart cells.

CHELATED MINERAL
A combo package of key
minerals like calcium and zinc,
as well as trace elements.

From Curatives to L-Carnitine Dietary supplements have come a long way since the herbal remedies of the 19th century.

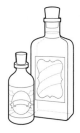 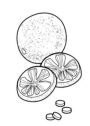 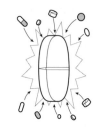 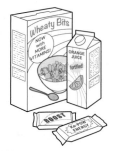

1800s
Some of the healing elixirs were little more than alcohol. Others contained more-harmful ingredients, like "the blue pill," or pilula hydrargyri, which combined mercury, glycerin, and licorice and was said to treat constipation.

1912
The Polish-born chemist Casimir Funk develops the concept of vitamins, or nonmineral nutrients for good health. He names the first one B1. By 1932, vitamin C is chemically identified as ascorbic acid.

1934
The multivitamin arrives and encounters skepticism amid rising sales. In the 1940s, a leading cardiologist calls the vitamin industry "the damnedest racket ever perpetrated upon the public."

1989
American physician Stephen DeFelice coins the term "nutraceutical" as energy bars and other foods enriched with vitamins are on the way to becoming a multibillion-dollar business.

revenue in 2011, which makes it one of the smaller players in the nutraceutical world. By comparison, GNC, a brand you may recognize from the mall, reported revenue of $2.07 billion. The world's largest pharmaceutical company, Pfizer, earned most of its $67 billion in 2011 sales from drugs, but it sold an estimated $1 billion in supplements like its Centrum vitamins.

The nutraceutical market is growing so fast among aging boomers that even giant food and drug companies are stumbling as they attempt to maintain their positions. In 2010, the Dannon Co., which makes Activia yogurt, settled allegations brought by 39 state attorneys general who objected to Activia ads suggesting the yogurt could prevent irregularity. A few weeks earlier, the drug company Bayer agreed to pay $3.3 million to three states after their attorneys general accused the company of claiming, wrongly, that one of its newer One a Day vitamin products reduces the risk of prostate cancer.

On the health form I completed for Usana, I reported my dietary habits (a combination of farmers market rectitude and late-night Rice Krispies Treats vice), sun exposure (less than 10 minutes a day), exercise routine (vigorous to the point of obsessive), and alcohol intake (enthusiastic). After I submitted the form, software at Usana crunched the data and kicked out a list of supplements I would need: eight pills in the morning and another eight at night, along with six other pills throughout the day. My a.m. HealthPak consisted of two Procosa IIs, two Mega Antioxidants, two Chelated Minerals, one CoQuinone 100, and one Proflavinol C 200.

One of the first things you learn about nutraceuticals is that the names are mostly made up. Procosa II is what Usana chose for a tablet that contains vitamin C bound with manganese and the chemical glucosamine sulfate, a naturally occurring compound found in the fluid around the joints that you can take as a supplement for arthritis. Usana's Mega Antioxidant pill contains vitamins A, B6, B12, C, D3, E, and K, along with 19 other ingredients.

What exactly are all these substances? I discovered that no government agency catalogs (let alone tests) dietary supplements. Under a 1994 law, the federal government defines dietary supplements as any vitamin, mineral, or herb (along with a few other more obscure substances) intended to be swallowed in order to augment diet. The U.S. Food and Drug Administration lacks the authority to approve prospective supplements for safety or effectiveness, and the agency can't act to restrict even a reputedly risky product until it hits the market. Since 1994, the FDA has banned only one dietary supplement—the alkaloid ephedrine, which can be used on its own as a weight-loss drug or as a precursor in the manufacture of crystal meth. Some critics of the supplement industry say the agency needs more power, but safety isn't the real problem with nutraceuticals, most of which do little except discharge with your urine. Instead, effectiveness is the issue: Many supplements may not do enough to be worth the money.

The makings of a guru

The decision whether to take nutraceuticals is complicated by the fact that the lines among the three categories—food, drug, and supplement—have always been scientifically blurry and politically contested. A century ago a Polish-born chemist named Casimir Funk coined the term "vitamine" in a paper about his work with a substance in the inner bran layer of rice that he labeled "B1" in an experiment. And so B1 became the first named vitamin. Without B1, later dubbed thiamine, humans develop a disease called beriberi, for which B1 pills can be a treatment. But is B1 a food (a part of rice), a drug (a cure for beriberi), or a supplement (an additive you take just in case)?

In the years after Funk's discovery, an industry was born. Even before World War II, doctors began recommending cod-liver oil because it could provide the newly discovered vitamins A and D. During the war, the military sent millions of dollars' worth of vitamin tablets to service members around the globe, and food companies bought vitamin powders to use as enrichments for not only bread but even beer and jelly. These "fortified" products were, in some ways, the first nutraceuticals.

Then, in the 1960s, the biochemist Linus Pauling began advocating controversial huge doses of vitamin C to prevent the common cold. Pauling—who had won two Nobel Prizes, one in 1954 for his chemistry research and one in 1962 for his antinuclear activism—had completed little rigorous research on the vitamin, but he had the makings of a guru. He was credentialed yet elfin, sympathetic yet persistent. Sales of vitamin C pills exploded after his blockbuster book *Vitamin C and the Common Cold* appeared in 1970. Pauling, who died in 1994 of prostate cancer at age 93, left a scientific legacy beyond his vitamin C crusade: the Linus Pauling Institute at Oregon State University, which provides a steady stream of peer-reviewed research into whether and how nutraceuticals work. The institute also produces many of the young nutritional scientists who go to work for the research departments of nutraceutical companies. When I visited Usana's Salt Lake City headquarters, it was a former Pauling student, a molecular biologist named Brian Dixon, who met with me to review my lab results.

Dixon is in his thirties, compact, and extremely polite. He wore jeans to our meeting, and he was unguarded as he gave me a tour of Usana's labs and warehouses. Usana manufactures 90% of its products at the Salt Lake City headquarters, which produces more than 22 million tablets each week. Like several other big supplement companies, Usana sells its products Avon-style, through networks of more than 200,000 independent distributors—husband-and-wife teams working from home, personal trainers looking for side money, unemployed people hoping for better. On my tour, I saw Usana's Wall of Fame, which is actually several walls along several hallways that display glossy head shots of the biggest vendors.

Direct selling from your home is a brutal way to make a living, one that requires unwavering conviction and optimism. That's why direct marketing is a perfect business model for nutraceuticals, a category of products based at least as much in hope as in data. And Usana, like several other major nutraceutical makers, is based in Utah, a state known for its faith and abstemiousness. When I asked for coffee on my visit to Usana, the PR team had to scramble to find an old coffee maker. Caffeine is frowned upon in the Mormon church.

Dixon and I reviewed copies of my two lab reports, including the baseline results from January and the post-regimen results from June. Each report showed 31 measurements, the first of which was "glucose, serum," a measure of my blood sugar: 83 milligrams per deciliter (mg/dl) in January and 88 mg/dl in June, a change neither statistically nor medically significant. In fact, even after more than 3,000 pills and a daily diet of fiber powders and protein bars, little had changed. Two measures of my kidney health (values for blood urea nitrogen and creatinine) were identical. Calcium, protein, sodium—none had varied much.

I asked two doctors to review my lab results: Braunstein at Cedars-Sinai and Stephen Dillon, my personal physician of 15 years. Both said only two of the values on my blood report had changed significantly. First, there was that 75% vitamin D increase, which the two of them attributed to the vitamin D3 supplement I had been taking (rather than to my spending more time outside). Second, my level of high-density lipoprotein (HDL) cholesterol—the good one— had leaped from 61 mg/dl in January to 89 mg/dl in June, an increase of 46%. Braunstein said he couldn't explain such a big surge. He pointed out that supplements that include niacin can amplify HDL cholesterol, but he suspected that my niacin dose of 40 mg per day was too low to account for such a large increase. Dillon speculated that the 2,000 mg of fish-oil concentrate I had been taking might have played a role.

I was frustrated by the lack of firm answers. When I asked Dixon what he thought about my HDL, he was careful. The FDA prohibits supplement companies from making unsupported health claims. "We make no representations that nutritional supplementation is a quick fix," he told me. "We just consider these nutritional supplements to be almost an insurance policy."

But health insurance of any kind isn't cheap. Usana billed TIME more than $1,200 for the five-month supply of nutraceuticals I took, although one of its direct sellers may have charged a client far more. (After this story appeared, Usana declined to accept payment. We returned hundreds of unused pills.) Braunstein said that for far less, Dillon could have done a simple blood test that would have shown my slightly-lower-than-normal vitamin D level. I could have then started buying over-the-counter, generic vitamin D tablets—and had money left over for a new gym membership.

Okay, but the supplements had also made me feel different—healthier, more robust. My blood hadn't changed, but a strong placebo response had occurred. I woke up every morning feeling vigorous in a way I hadn't in years. And that turned out to be a problem.

The licensing effect

One morning in March, a couple of months into my nutraceutical regimen, I noticed that my jeans were tight. A week later, I went up a notch on my belt. Usana had asked me to keep a health log, and now I looked back. I was 170 pounds on Feb. 1, 175 pounds by late February, and 180 on March 30.

I had also been recording my meals. I was eating fine in early February. On Feb. 6, for instance, I had grilled chicken, vegetables, and brown rice for dinner, along with pineapple juice. But the following month, there were entries like this one, for March 2: "Burger, a few fries, and onion rings." That came after an afternoon chocolate croissant.

Psychologists have a name for my behavior: the licensing effect. (Nutritionists have called it compensation.) The nutraceuticals had made me feel virtuous. Vitamin C? Niacin? Vitamin K? I had plenty. Any nutrient that my body could possibly need would be provided by these pills and powders. So I changed my routine. Other people may have to eat sautéed kale, but I get fries. (A study published in the journal *Addiction* shows that the same thing happened with smokers: Those who took pills they believed were vitamins—the pills were actually just sugar— smoked significantly more cigarettes afterward than those in a control group.)

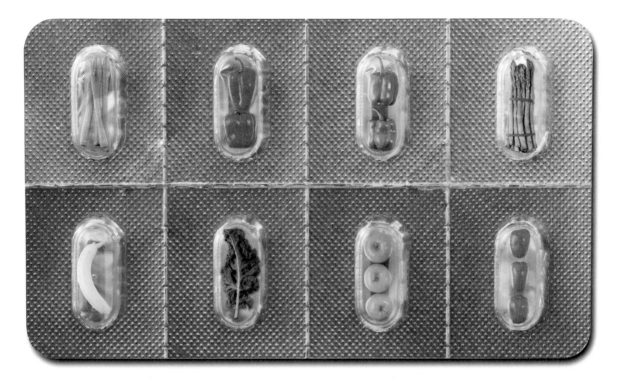

It took me three months to lose the weight. In the end, Dixon helped me do it. He emphasized that his company's products should be taken only in concert with a nutritious diet and plenty of exercise, water, and sleep. He also sent me a cookbook, *Low-Glycemic Meals in Minutes*; the meals were better than they sound.

Dixon was always a meticulous scientist, but then I thought about how most Usana products are sold, through networks of non-experts, all those homemakers trying to get on the Wall of Fame. Would they be as scrupulous about recommending Usana products only as an adjunct to a healthy diet? Usana's annual meetings, which draw thousands of enthusiastic sellers to convention centers around the country, can seem more like tent revivals than scientific conclaves. Nutraceuticals may or may not make people healthy, but those who sell and consume them can become zealous believers in health.

And yet some doctors worry that nutraceutical enthusiasts will come to believe that if a little vitamin help is good, more will be better. Vitamin overdose is rare, though Eduardo Marbán, director of the Cedars-Sinai Heart Institute, has found that extreme doses of antioxidants can cause genetic mutations in stem cells. He says he virtually never recommends supplements. "I

think a normal diet would suffice in every case that I know of," he told me. "And I'm worried about the little old lady who takes 20 vitamin pills a day." Marbán's deep skepticism about nutraceuticals has a long history in the medical community. In the 1940s, Ernst Boas, a famous Columbia University cardiologist, called the vitamin business "the damnedest racket ever perpetrated upon the public."

That's going a bit far—but the aura of snake oil persuaded me, eventually, to toss my remaining pills and fiber powder (though I think Usana's Nutrimeal shakes are a delicious breakfast). People ask me all the time whether I felt different when I was taking the pills and if I feel different now that I have stopped.

I don't wake up now with that feeling of the lion who will eat the world. But I make better food choices. On nutraceuticals, I had come to believe that health could be a set of tablets to take rather than a series of responsibilities to meet—water instead of soda, an apple instead of chips, real fish instead of a giant fish-oil capsule. You can take vitamins on the faith that they will make you better—and if you have a real vitamin deficiency, they will. But there's more science behind another way of getting your vitamins: eating right.

A version of this story originally appeared in TIME *magazine.*

All About
The Essentials

From vitamin A to zinc, a look at some of the scientific lore about the substances you can't live without.

Vitamin and mineral supplements continue to spark some debate: Who should take them? How much should you take? But one fact isn't in dispute: Good health depends on each of the 13 vitamins and 16 essential minerals. The best way to get them, of course, is with a well-rounded diet that is heavy on whole foods and light on the processed kind. But for many people, children and the elderly especially, regular or occasional supplements may be the next best thing. Here's some other essential—or at least interesting—info about vitamins and minerals.

VITAMIN K, which gets its name from the German for "coagulation," does exactly that: thickens blood. Doctors may recommend vitamin K, found in kale and other green vegetables, to patients who have been taking a blood thinner before certain surgeries to reduce the risk of bleeding.

After calcium, **PHOSPHORUS** is the most abundant mineral in the body and, along with calcium, is the foundation of bones and teeth. It is present in soybeans and avocados, as well as in many other foods, and assists most metabolic actions, including kidney function and cell growth.

At the beginning of the 20th century, various scientists determined that unpolished rice prevented beriberi but polished rice did not. Their conclusion—that something crucial lurked in the husk—was the first step in the **DISCOVERY OF VITAMINS.**

Many synthetic vitamins act very much like their natural counterparts, but that is not the case with **VITAMIN E.** Natural E has a different molecular shape, making it easier to absorb and thus more beneficial to the body. Best known as an antioxidant, it comes from nuts, spinach, and oils.

VITAMIN D exists in only a few foods—oily fish, mostly—which is why dairy owners add it to their milk. Most younger people get enough from sunshine. As we age, though, our skin is less able to convert sunshine into vitamin D. In fact, recent studies suggest a lot more people are D deficient than previously thought. Supplement users, read the label: vitamin D3 is more effective than D2.

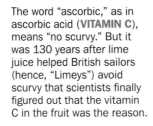

The word "ascorbic," as in ascorbic acid (**VITAMIN C**), means "no scurvy." But it was 130 years after lime juice helped British sailors (hence, "Limeys") avoid scurvy that scientists finally figured out that the vitamin C in the fruit was the reason.

THE EIGHT B VITAMINS were once all thought to be a singular entity. Turns out that while they often occur in the same foods—meat, whole grains, vegetables—they are chemically distinct. Most are well known by other names: B3, for instance, is niacin, found in chicken and mushrooms; B9 is folic acid, found in leafy vegetables and egg yolks. Exceptions to the name rule are B6, found in bananas, and B12, found in seafood. After just three weeks of a diet lacking in thiamine (B1), which is found in fish and soybeans, the first signs of deficiency begin to reveal themselves. Fatigue and memory loss come first. Down the line? Brain deterioration.

We need to think about getting enough of the water-soluble vitamins—**C AND THE EIGHT Bs**—every day, but not the fat-soluble vitamins (A, D, E, and K). Because they aren't flushed from the system so easily, they can reach toxic levels if we overdo it. Eating a polar bear's liver can be fatal because it is so packed with vitamin A.

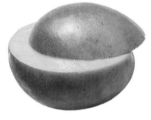

Of the 16 minerals that are generally considered essential, only the **SEVEN MACROMINERALS**—calcium, chlorine, magnesium, phosphorous, potassium, sodium, and sulfur—are needed in more than trace amounts. In fact, other minerals can be toxic in more than small doses. For instance, too much fluoride—from, say, more than a gallon of black tea a day—can cause brittle bones and an increased risk of fracture.

TOO LITTLE VITAMIN A, found in fruits such as mangoes as well as most vegetables and liver (polar bear and otherwise), can cause night blindness, dry skin, and an increased risk of infection. An estimated 10% of pregnant women around the world have dry-eye syndrome from vitamin-A deficiency.

Anecdotal evidence suggests that **VITAMIN B5** (pantothenic acid) might help prevent gray hair and wrinkles. You can get what you need of it in cauliflower, kale, and beef. Other popular vitamins for hair health include A (to prevent loss) and E (to encourage growth).

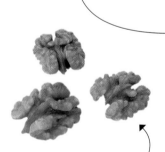

IRON IS A TRACE MINERAL, meaning that we need fewer than 5 grams a day. Less than that can cause fatigue and anemia. To get enough, eat your beans. On the other hand, too much zinc, another trace mineral, can suppress the immune system. Zinc is found in nuts.

IRON SUPPLEMENTS are absorbed much better when taken together with vitamin C, and absorbed much more poorly when taken with calcium. Calcium, by the way, also prevents the absorption of some prescription drugs, including most thyroid medicines. Always do your research before taking pills in combination.

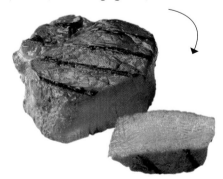

Graphic designed by Anne-Michelle Gallero

Does God Want You To Be Thin?

A Bible passage inspired Pastor Rick Warren's congregation to lose a collective 260,000 pounds. How faith can fight obesity. **By Jeffrey Kluger & Elizabeth Dias**

"HAVE YOU HUGGED A PASTOR TODAY?" HE ASKS AS HE ENTERS A ROOM. "It's good for your health." And it does seem that way, since to share a hug with Warren is to be gathered into a big, benign, bearish embrace—a feeling that makes you hope he never loses another ounce.

But Warren, 58, once weighed 295 pounds—90 pounds too much for his 6-foot 3-inch frame—and still needs to drop another 35 pounds to reach a healthy weight. It hasn't taken him all that long to lose as much as he has; he began getting fit only in the past 18 months, which is an awful lot less time than it took him to get fat. "I've only put on three pounds a year," he tells the members of his evangelical Saddleback Church in Lake Forest, Calif. "But I've been your pastor for 30 years."

Nearly everything about Warren is big. Saddleback has a stunning 20,000 weekly attendees across 10 campuses. He is the author of multiple books, including *The Purpose Driven Life*, the bestselling nonfiction hardback in American history—after

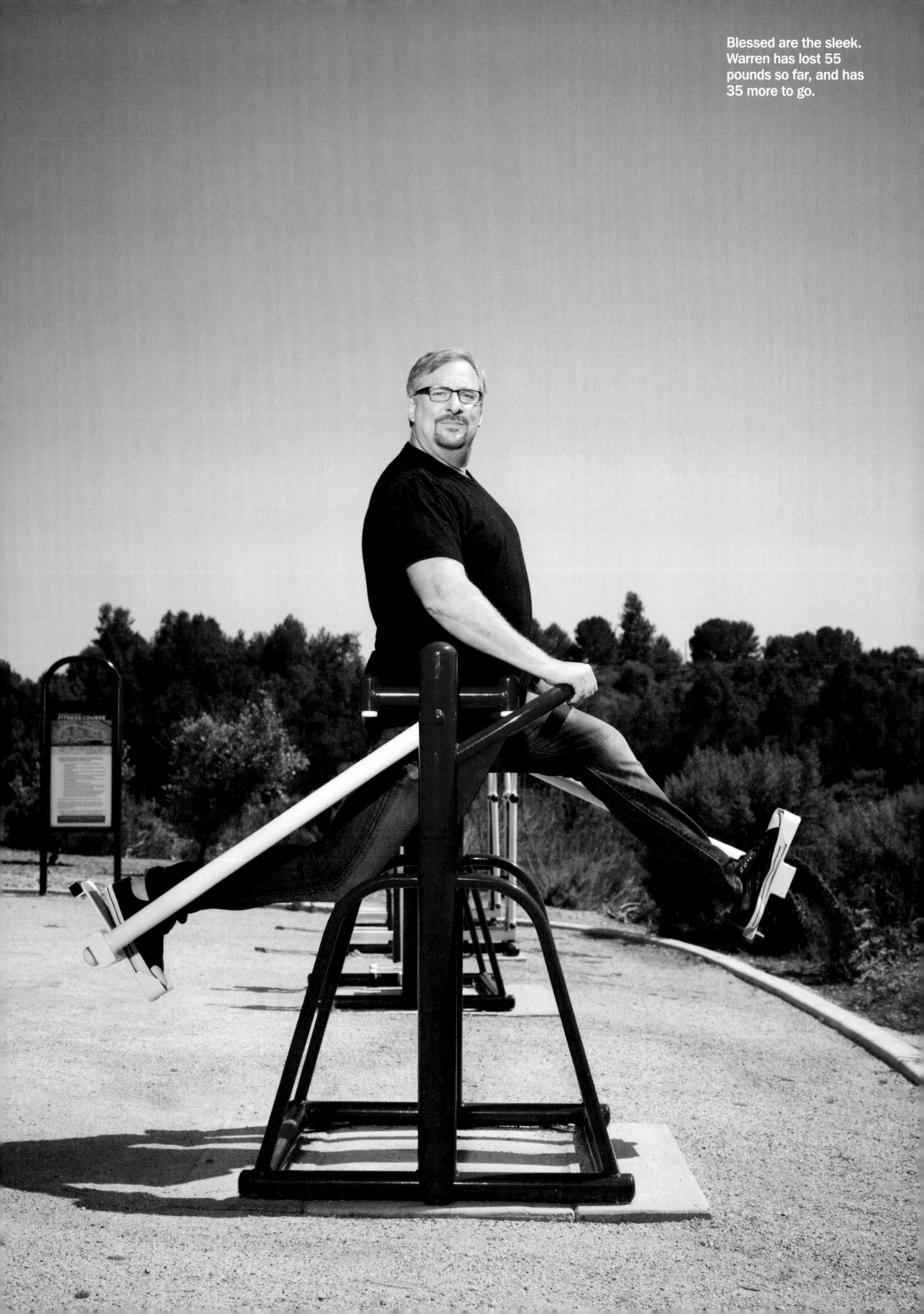

Blessed are the sleek. Warren has lost 55 pounds so far, and has 35 more to go.

the Bible, appropriately—with 32 million copies in print worldwide and editions published in 97 languages. He gave the invocation at the 2009 presidential Inauguration and interviewed candidates Barack Obama and John McCain, one on one, on national TV in 2008, a gig most news anchors would have killed to land.

But in 2010, Warren discovered a problem in his church. It was after a high-volume baptism session, when he and other Saddleback pastors administered the sacrament to some 800 congregants in less than four hours. That's three people per minute, and since Warren prefers to baptize by immersion, he wound up having to dip and lift a whole lot of cumulative weight.

"Man, we're all fat," he recalls thinking.

And so they were. As the church members later learned, the average weight of Saddleback women was 170 pounds, and it was 210 pounds for men—which meant Warren and the others immersed 160,000 pounds of very unhealthy humanity that day. Before the ceremony was even over, he decided to do something about the problem. The answer, he believed, lay in the Book of Daniel.

One of the 39 books of the Old Testament, Daniel tells the story of four Jewish boys who were taken to the court of the conquering King Nebuchadnezzar to be trained and fed in the royal manner so that they might serve in the

True Believers Nine Daniel Plan enthusiasts describe its impact on their lives.

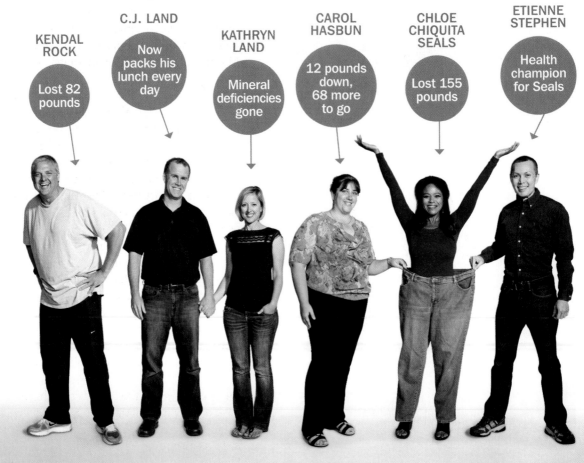

KENDAL ROCK — Lost 82 pounds

C.J. LAND — Now packs his lunch every day

KATHRYN LAND — Mineral deficiencies gone

CAROL HASBUN — 12 pounds down, 68 more to go

CHLOE CHIQUITA SEALS — Lost 155 pounds

ETIENNE STEPHEN — Health champion for Seals

King's palace. The boys, led by Daniel, accepted the King's teaching but would go nowhere near the King's table, refusing to defile themselves with the meat and wine he offered them. They chose vegetables and water instead—and grew fitter and finer for their efforts.

Warren's congregants were moving in precisely the opposite direction, and Americans in general have been doing the same: Two-thirds of adults in the U.S. are overweight or obese, as are up to one-third of children. More than 20% of all adolescents have diabetes or pre-diabetes, up from 9% in 2000. Portion sizes and waistlines are out of control, and the current generation of kids is on track to be the first in American history to be less healthy than their parents.

Warren reckoned that he was in a position to help change all that. On Jan. 15, 2011, he launched the Daniel Plan, a sweeping health-and-fitness program for Saddleback members that begins with a commonsense diet of 70% unprocessed fruits and vegetables and 30% lean protein, whole grains, and starchy vegetables. The plan includes exercise groups, nutrition training, sports, recipe tips, small support-group meetings, Walk and Worship sessions, and more.

Warren and his team expected perhaps 200 people to sign up after the kickoff rally, but 6,000 did, with another 1,200 joining online—a number that has risen to 15,000. The church has lost a collective 260,000 pounds in the past year, and Warren jokes that he's shooting for the equivalent of a jumbo jet (800,000 pounds, for the record, fully fueled and loaded). A man with Warren's profile attracts other big names, and Mehmet Oz, Daniel Amen, and Mark Hyman—a cardiologist, a neurologist, and a nutritionist (and significantly, of Muslim, Christian, and Jewish roots)—have volunteered their time to the cause.

You don't have to be a cynic to observe that diet plans that make and at first support extraordinary claims are not new. But you don't have to be a person of faith—any faith—to admit that a wellness plan based at least in part on Scripture seems fresher. A robust body of scientific evidence supports a link between faith and health. Attendance at religious services has been shown to add two to three years to life, for example. You may believe that there's something divine in that; you may believe that it's simply the proven ability of any group to improve the welfare of all its members. Either way, you can't argue with the results.

"The community is the cure," says Hyman. "The group is the medicine. There are feedback loops, accountability, support."

Those are all things Warren's church serves up—along with a very generous helping of evangelical Christianity. The central belief that drives the Daniel Plan is best captured by a T-shirt many of the participants wear that reads, "God created it/ Jesus died for it/ The Holy Spirit lives in it/ Shouldn't you take care of it?" The "it," of course,

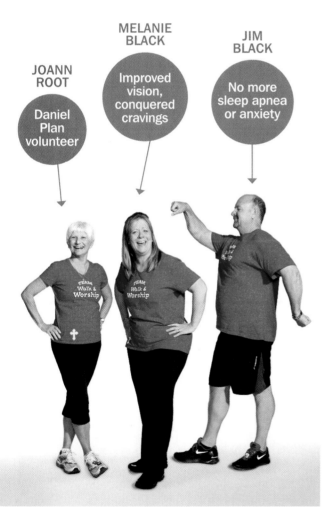

JOANN ROOT

Daniel Plan volunteer

MELANIE BLACK

Improved vision, conquered cravings

JIM BLACK

No more sleep apnea or anxiety

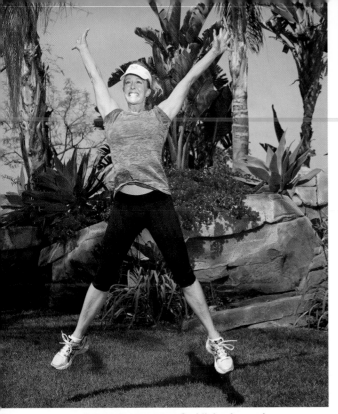

THE GOOD WORKOUT Saddleback member Juli Cuccia attends weekly sessions.

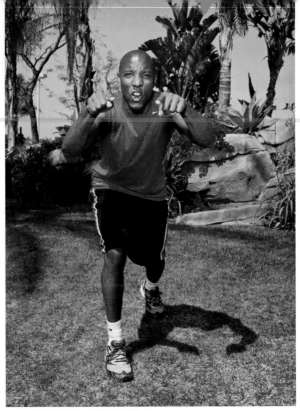

PRAISE THE SWEAT Trainer Tony Lattimore leads free boot-camp classes.

is the body, and evangelicals teach that it's not yours at all. Instead, our bodies are gifts from God, and we are expected to return them in the best shape possible. Just as some religious communities found their way to environmentalism through the idea that we are only stewards of the earth, so too must we remember that we are not the sole owners of our flesh.

"My body is not my own. My body is on loan," says Jim Black, a physical therapist who joined the program with his wife, Melanie. "I have to give it back."

The Book of Daniel does not actually prescribe a diet to help us look after ourselves. "Nowhere in the Bible does it say, 'This is what they should eat,'" says C.L. Seow, a Daniel scholar and professor at Princeton Theological Seminary. The critical passage, he explains, has to do with resistance, with a rejection of privilege. "The point is the triumph of God."

Even the sins of gluttony and vanity—dieting's opposite poles—have no real role in the Daniel Plan. "That doesn't reflect my heart," says Dee Eastman, a Saddleback member and the director of the Daniel Plan. Instead, she explains, it is about freeing people from shame or illness so that they can fulfill God's plan for them. God does not necessarily want you to be thin, but he very much wants you to be healthy.

All this works well on the Saddleback campus, but Warren has dreams of taking the plan wide— to 1 billion people around the world in the next decade, says Hyman. That means either recruiting and converting a great many new members or finding what's scalable and nondenominational in the program and getting it out to a global population that's getting fatter, slower, and sicker all the time.

Bodies on loan

It was just 16 months ago that Chloe Chiquita Seals decided to change her life—and it badly needed changing. At 270 pounds, she spent most of her time in her house, too self-conscious to leave. "I was a hermit," she says. "I was afraid to go out, to walk down the street." Seals didn't have much, but she did have a friend—Etienne Stephen, a Saddleback member she had known since college. He encouraged her to attend the Daniel Plan kickoff rally, and she signed up for the program straightaway.

More important than simply introducing Seals to the program, Stephen has also guided her through it. Daniel Plan participants are encouraged to form small groups with only five or so members, led by what the church calls a champion. Currently about 5,000 such groups meet regularly, and they are the true core of the program. Stephen takes his role as Seals's champion seriously—helping her make food substitutions, teaching her to read supermarket labels, even paying for a gym membership for her.

The plan has worked extraordinarily well for Seals so far: She has lost half her body weight and gone from a size 22 to a size 2. And in the spirit of the pay-it-forward fellowship that the Daniel Plan is designed to foster, she has recruited Carol Hasbun, a friend of four years' standing who has been in the program for about a month. Seals has helped her shop, taught her to make healthy pizza, gone through her kitchen cabinets, and, following a Daniel Plan video, cleaned out all the nasty stuff.

"My goal is to lose 80 pounds," Hasbun says, "hopefully in a year or two years." Seals is quick to back her up. "You are going to get there," she says.

By keeping the menu interesting, the Daniel Plan makes such an ambitious goal easier to reach. Cooking classes and recipe tips, which are offered on the Saddleback campus and online, include dishes like agave-glazed-salmon tacos in blue-corn tortillas with poblano-and-avocado lime sauce, accompanied by napa cabbage slaw—weighing in at just 370 calories.

It would be easy if the Daniel Plan called on its members to do nothing more than meet, shop, and cook, but it's a decidedly more vigorous regimen than that. On a recent Sunday morning, 60 people had already shown up on the campus for a 9 a.m. boot-camp class, led by Tony Lattimore, a church member and personal trainer. Lattimore's usual rate is $75 per hour, but his Saddleback classes are free. "We live completely on faith," says his wife, Kimberly.

Nearby, a volleyball game is going on at the community center and restaurant known as the Refinery—recalling the biblical passages that refer to God's refining power. The building also has a basketball court and Frisbee golf course, and outdoor lights are in the works so that members can play at night. An organic garden has been planted, and the harvest is used in the restaurant and in the food pantry that helps feed the needy. Not all the fare in the restaurant is healthy (Warren believes the program should neither be nor feel mandatory), but each selection does bear a green, yellow, or red star indicating the degree of caution church members should exercise before choosing it.

Even doctors who don't agree with the religious element of the plan would find it hard to dispute that the overall regimen is well designed—and that this kind of program is badly needed everywhere. "By the end of this decade, there will be 50 million people per year dying worldwide from chronic, lifestyle-related diseases, compared with 20 million dying from infectious diseases," says Hyman. "These are things we could be preventing."

Taking it wide

If churches can be a solution to the obesity problem, they also, in some ways, helped create it. Amen was a devout Christian long before he became involved with the Daniel Plan. He recalls a day in 2010 when he entered the church he regularly attended and found doughnuts for sale and hot dogs and sausages cooking outside while the minister talked about the ice cream festival held the night before. Amen began scrawling notes to himself: "They have no idea they are sending people to heaven early. This has got to change."

He began praying for guidance, and just two

VEGGIE TALES Daniel Plan director Dee Eastman at Saddleback's organic farm

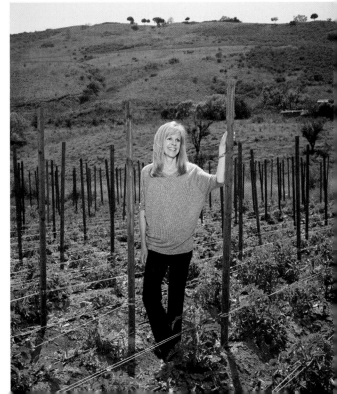

For God and Waistline
What the Daniel Plan tells its followers.

1. Connect for success
Talk with a doctor and learn your overall health status, including your measurements. Get the bad foods out of your pantry, and above all, join a small support group at your church.

2. Rely on God's power
Find encouragement from Bible passages like this one from the New Testament: "I can do all things through Christ, who gives me strength."

3. Eat delicious whole foods
Follow the 70/30 rule: 70% of a daily diet should consist of whole foods like raw or lightly cooked vegetables, fruits, nuts, and seeds, while 30% is for lean protein, whole grains, and starchy vegetables.

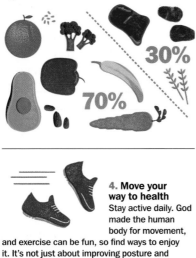

30%

70%

4. Move your way to health
Stay active daily. God made the human body for movement, and exercise can be fun, so find ways to enjoy it. It's not just about improving posture and flexibility; build in hikes with friends and after-dinner swims.

5. Think sharper and smarter
Get at least seven to eight hours of sleep per night. Deep breathing and exercise will help reduce stress. Avoid brain robbers like alcohol, drugs, cigarettes, cigars, and concussion-causing sports. Adding certain spices to your food can stimulate your brain. (Sage may boost memory, and cinnamon may increase attention.) When negative thoughts pop into your head, replace them with Scripture.

6. Heal for life
The Daniel Plan is a lifestyle, not a diet. The point is long-term abundance, not deprivation. Sugar addictions and food cravings trigger overeating, often leading to chronic diseases. Like Daniel before the conquering King, refuse to compromise.

weeks later Warren called and asked him to participate in the Daniel Plan. "I'm thinking, No way," Amen says. "God does not usually answer my prayer that fast and in a big way."

Warren's idea of keeping the church in the game but using it to fix rather than create problems appealed to Amen, in part because it's applicable to all faiths. There's nothing that says a mosque can't have exercise classes and cooking demonstrations; there's nothing that says a synagogue can't have a website and small-group support. Other churches are already clamoring for the Daniel Plan, and a friend of Warren's who is a rabbi wants to offer the plan in his synagogue.

Tapping the church as an existing root system for health can be used in an even bigger way in the developing world, something that's central to a newly launched mission Warren calls the PEACE Plan, an acronym for planting churches around the world, equipping leaders, assisting the poor, caring for the sick, and educating the next genera-

tion. A beta test for the PEACE Plan occurred in 2005, when Paul Kagame, President of Rwanda, moved by the message of *The Purpose Driven Life*, contacted Warren and told him he wanted to create a purpose-driven country.

Saddleback volunteers traveled to Rwanda and saw that while there were just three large hospitals in one province, there were 869 churches, most of which could do double duty as clinics and care stations. Today 4,000 church-affiliated volunteers have been mobilized in Rwanda, providing screening for HIV/AIDS and hypertension and initiating feeding, clean-water, education, and adoption programs. Saddleback is focusing on a dozen other cities around the world—including Amman, Johannesburg, Moscow, Tokyo, and Mexico City—for the access they provide to local disadvantaged populations. The Daniel Plan might actually have a role in the PEACE Plan too, since even in desperately poor places, cheap, processed Western-style fare has wreaked havoc on health. "Eighty percent of all diabetics are in the developing world," says Amen. "The commercial used to say, 'I'd like to buy the world a Coke.' Well, I guess we did."

Is it for everyone?

There's no guarantee that the Daniel Plan, innovative as it is, will move the health needle over the long term. Diet plans have an extraordinary failure rate for a great many reasons. A daunting mix of habit, genetics, and even addictive behavior drive obesity, as does simple metabolism: The earlier in life you become fat, the more you change the way you process food.

And yet there's no denying the hand-in-glove way that faith and health mix. People who attend services have a lower risk of dying in any one year than people who don't. Studies have shown that belief in a loving God as opposed to a punishing God is linked to faster recovery after surgery. People with HIV/AIDS tend to do better when they belong to a religious community. One study even found that church members who give service have better health profiles than those who receive service—confirming that it truly does pay to care for others. The precise mechanism behind these findings—divinity, biology, or both—matters less than the fact that the benefits are real.

But the plan could face other obstacles. One of the things that make an evangelical health program so easy to take in nonevangelical communities is Warren's singular style. There's a hint of good-natured mischief to him, which nicely leavens the messages he delivers about such profound issues as life, death, and afterlife. He takes an almost teenlike pleasure in talking about his Twitter feed and then adds, "You know, if you don't follow me on Twitter, you'll go to hell."

The line gets the intended laugh, but the fact is, hell does remain part of his teachings. "You have friends who don't know Jesus," he has told his followers. "You know people who are headed to hell." That may be a common evangelical belief, but it fits uneasily with the no-judgments ethos of the Daniel Plan.

The plan's website also makes clear that for all the multicultural character of the program, there is a line that will not be crossed. The Frequently Asked Questions section of the site explains that while doctors of other faiths are part of the plan, they "are helping us as friends," and the church will never compromise its belief that "Jesus is the only way to heaven or that the Bible is the 100% completely infallible and perfect word of God."

And while the idea that your body is on loan can be a nice motivator if you want to lose weight, it can be just as powerful a tool to regulate—and proscribe—sexual behavior. "You don't have the right to just share your body with anyone!" says one piece of Daniel Plan material that addresses sexuality. Perhaps unsurprisingly, Warren has earned the wrath of the gay community for his opposition to same-sex marriage, though he has not belabored the issue.

All the same, it would be more than a little disingenuous for outsiders to profess themselves shocked—shocked!—that an evangelical church believes in heaven, hell, and a literal interpretation of the Bible and has a rule or two about human sexuality. You can hardly walk into a vegan restaurant and then get mad when you can't order a burger.

More important, unlike evangelical teachings as a whole, the Daniel Plan can easily be taken cafeteria-style. Embrace what it has to say about the power of community and the responsibility of caring for the only body you'll ever have, fold in some of your own religion if you choose, and leave the rest. Hyman, who likes to laugh about how a Jewish doctor from New York wound up partnering with Warren, thinks about this a lot. "Community-based models work," he says. "I go on *The 700 Club*, and people ask me why I appear with Pat Robertson. But we all get sick, regardless of religion. We have bodies, we care about our children and about creating a healthier world."

That's not a bad goal—and harnessing the power, commitment, and organizational skills of the faith-based community is not a bad way to get there. It's not the only way, but no one says it has to be. You may or may not believe in heaven, but good health, long life, and fellowship do feel like a little slice of it.

A version of this story originally appeared in TIME *magazine.*

10 Foods You Can't Get Enough Of

Okay, that's not quite true: Too much of anything can get you in trouble. In particular, nuts are packed with fat—the good fat, sure, but fat all the same. Yet if you build your diet around the following foods, you will be doing your body a big favor, says Donald Hensrud, medical editor of *The Mayo Clinic Diet*. And don't panic when you don't see whipped cream on the list; there's always room for a splurge. (In fact, a little chocolate—preferably dark—every now and then may actually confer some benefit.) "It's what we eat the majority of the time that influences our health," Hensrud says. The terrific 10:

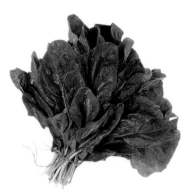

1. Spinach
Actually, any leafy green— dark lettuce, kale, baby bok choy—all are loaded with nutrients and very low in calories. And that's an unbeatable combination.

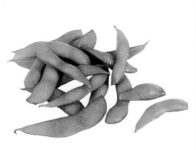

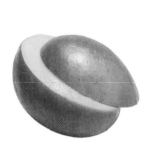

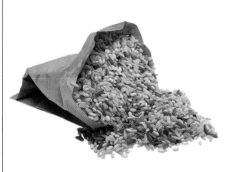

5. Soybeans
As good a protein source as there is—better, really, because soybeans contain little fat and no cholesterol, making them the thinking person's red meat substitute.

6. Mango
Fruits in general are a great low-calorie way to satisfy a sweet tooth, and the antioxidant compounds found in mangoes may help protect against certain cancers. Also, their relatively high-fiber content helps lower cholesterol.

7. Brown rice
Whole grains, of which brown rice is among the best, are good sources of complex carbohydrates and key vitamins and minerals. Also low in fat, they've been linked to a lower risk of heart disease, diabetes, cancers, and other health problems.

*Graphic designed by
Anne-Michelle Gallero*

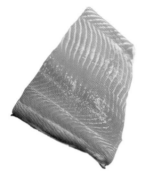

2. Salmon

All fish are good protein sources, of course, but if you eat just one kind this week, make it this one. Salmon is particularly high in heart-healthy omega-3 fatty acids as well.

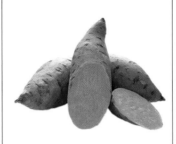

3. Sweet potatoes

These colorful tubers are high in the antioxidant beta carotene, which your body converts to vitamin A, and vitamin A may reduce the risk of some cancers. Sweet potatoes are a good source of fiber, vitamin B6, and potassium too. Also, half a large one has fewer than 100 calories.

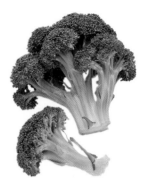

4. Broccoli

Besides being a good source of folate, which can lower the risk of some diseases and promote red blood cell production, broccoli contains isothiocyanates and other many-syllabled compounds that may help prevent heart disease, diabetes, and some cancers. Bonus: It's an excellent source of vitamin C.

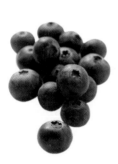

8. Blueberries

First among their berry equals, blueberries are a bit higher in antioxidants and other phytonutrients that may help prevent chronic diseases. But all berries are a low-calorie source of fiber and vitamin C as well.

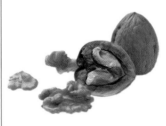

9. Walnuts

Other nuts can reduce cholesterol too, but what separates walnuts from the crowd is their significant amount of omega-3 fatty acids.

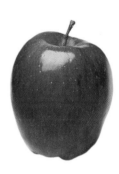

10. Apples

You didn't think the old rhyme was a lie, did you? Apples are a good source of pectin, a soluble fiber that can lower cholesterol and glucose levels. And they're a good source of vitamin C.

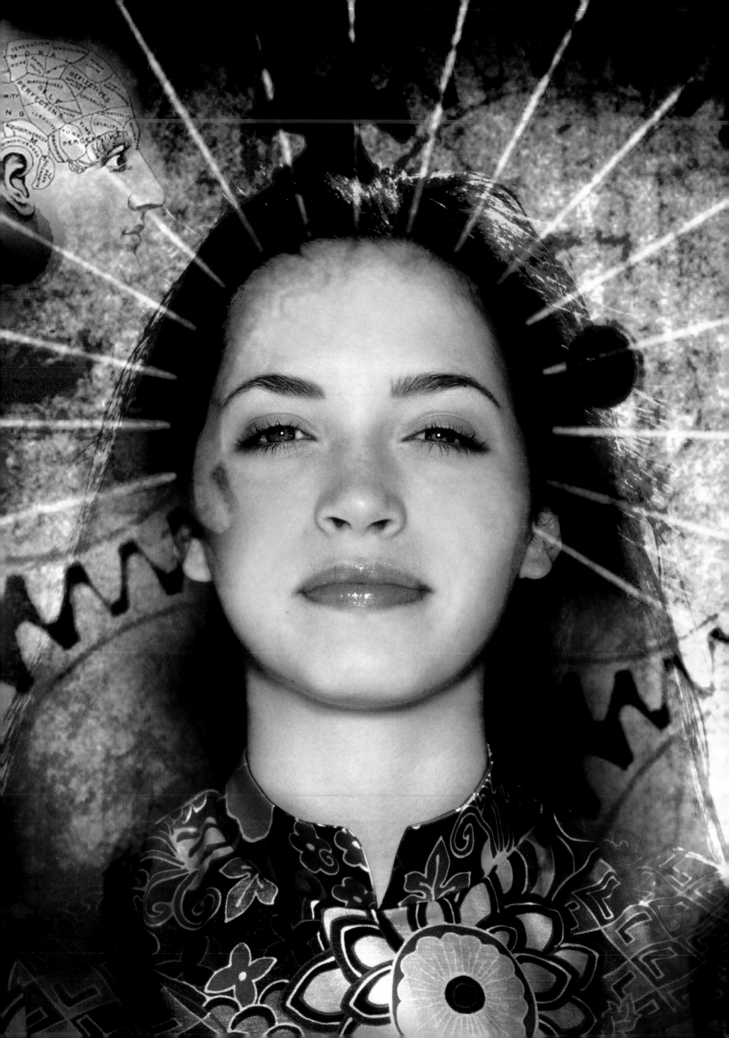

Empowering
Your Mind

The Magic of The Placebo

Neuroscience is finding a world of insights—and healing—in the lowly sugar pill. **By David Bjerklie**

THE STUDIES HARDLY SEEM A SHINING EXAMPLE OF MEDICINE'S HEALING grace. Patients suffering pain, depression, and even Parkinson's disease are treated with sugar pills, saline injections, or sham surgery. Irritable-bowel sufferers are given fake acupuncture. Women with polycystic ovarian syndrome, a common cause of infertility, are prescribed bogus remedies. But these "treatments" aren't the latest outrages of medical malfeasance. In fact, the subjects felt better, coped better, moved better, experienced fewer symptoms, even conceived better. What in the name of Hippocrates is going on here?

You have just entered the funhouse world of placebos. The supervised deceptions listed above are actually recent, scrupulously conducted research trials designed to investigate the healing power of the mind. Traditionally, the accepted role of placebos is to serve as inactive controls in randomized clinical studies, the baseline yardstick by which scientific discipline and objectivity are ensured and results measured. But

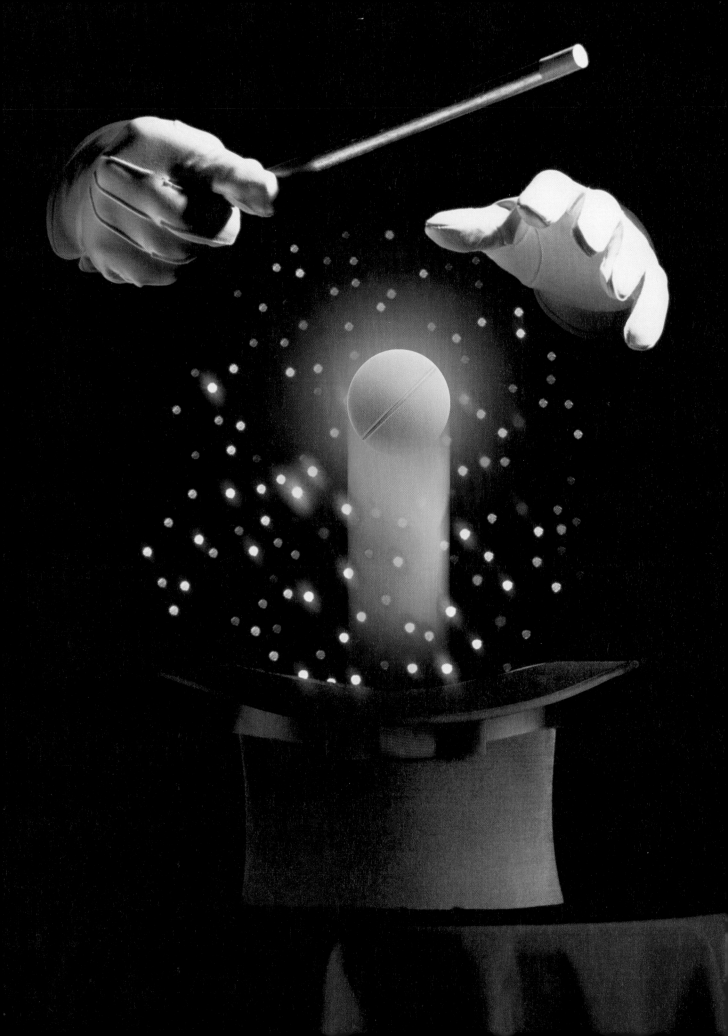

increasingly, placebos are also the rising stars of their own branch of research, one that seeks to understand the power of potions and procedures that, by all rights, should be completely ineffectual.

For generations, caregivers doled out versions of the classic placebo—an inert sugar or starch pill—as a passive token of hope and compassion. They were offered to patients who desperately wanted some sort of treatment when none was available or called for. These days placebos are commonly vitamins or over-the-counter analgesics rather than sugar pills, but their purpose is the same. This is why a patient who isn't feeling quite up to par might end up with a prescription for vitamin B12. Even a bona fide medicine can be a placebo if it is offered in minute doses or for conditions that aren't likely to respond to it. And the practice is more common than most patients might suspect (a recent survey of U.S. internists and rheumatologists found that some 50% regularly prescribe placebos).

The use of placebos is widespread for good reason. As it turns out, placebos are "much more powerful" than previously imagined, according to Fabrizio Benedetti of the University of Turin in Italy. Not only is the placebo effect real, says Benedetti, but "it is also a melting pot of neuroscientific concepts and ideas" that raises questions about psychology and physiology, not to mention challenges to current medical practices.

Placebos (Latin for "I shall please") are most commonly defined in terms of what they lack: active ingredients. But that is exactly the wrong way to look at them. "Placebos are not inert substances," wrote Benedetti and his colleagues in a recent paper. "They are made of words and rituals, symbols and meanings, and all these elements are active in shaping the patient's brain." And although the neuroscience is new, the knowledge that the mind can fool the body into feeling better has been a go-to secret of healers for millennia.

What has changed today is our modern need to put a label on that process, says Jon Tilburt of Mayo Clinic. Doctors are trained to want cause-and-effect explanations. They want to be able to define the mechanisms of improvement, to see "something" rather than "nothing." But most patients, says Tilburt, whose research focuses on relationships and values in medicine, "are pragmatists, not ideologues. They want to feel better, and they don't much care how that is achieved." Placebos represent one of the paths by which patients have always come to feel better. Call that path what you will, says Tilburt, "but it is definitely not nothing."

How do placebos work?

Neuroscientists, on the other hand, are eager to dive into the complexities of those pathways. The key to understanding the mysteries of placebos, says Benedetti, author most recently of *The Patient's Brain*, is that there is not one effect, but many. And to understand that, it's first important to recognize what placebos are not. Some people get better by themselves. Some seem to improve because they initially appeared to be sicker than they really were. And sometimes both patients and doctors kid themselves into seeing improvement when there isn't any. Spontaneous remission, testing error, wishful thinking … these are not placebo effects. Real placebo effects are genuine psychobiological phenomena in the brain that produce measurable changes in the body.

Consider the clout of expectation. What we experience depends partly on what we expect to experience, consciously or not. "Expectations," says psychologist Jane Metrik of Brown University's Center for Alcohol and Addiction Studies, "help us to recognize and classify all sorts of stimuli. There is great survival value in that." Healing value too. Expectations can activate the same neurochemical pathways triggered by our pursuit of food, water, and sex. They can also drive the body's ebb and flow of stress hormones. In short, expectations produce real, physiological change, often at the speed of thought. And it doesn't matter that those expectations might be activated by a sugar pill. When a placebo works it doesn't mean a patient's symptoms—say, pain, depression, or anxiety—aren't real. It just means that the neurochemical changes produced by the expectation of relief are just as real.

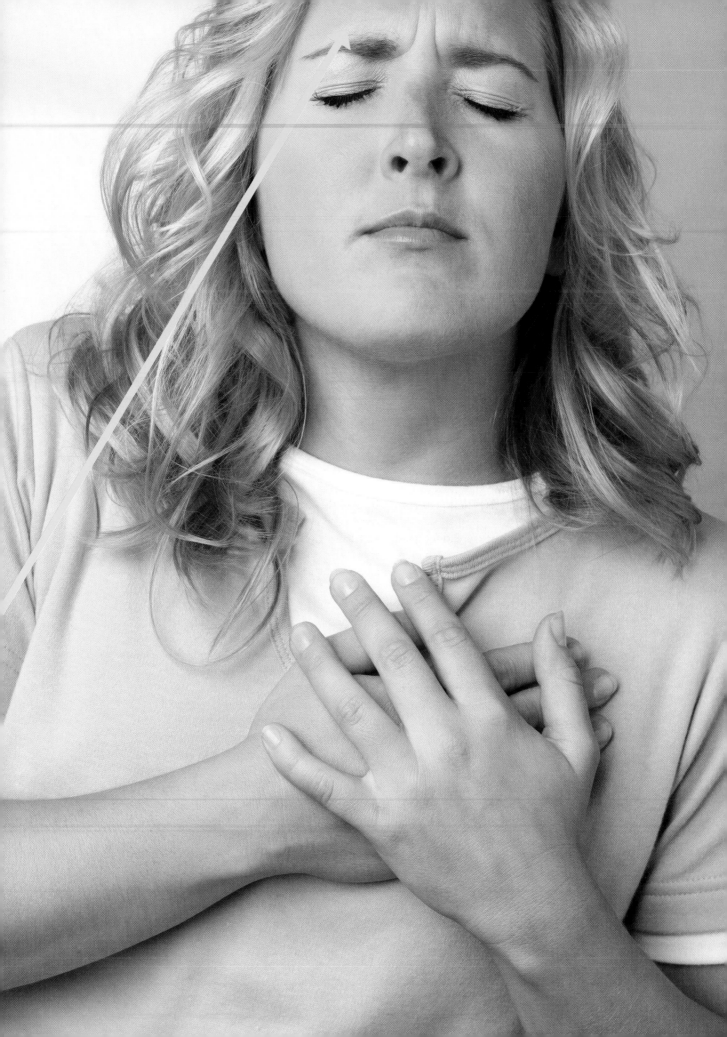

Doctors can use expectations to their advantage, even when they are administering potent drugs. Here's a scenario that plays out in emergency rooms every day. "If a patient needs pain medicine, I make sure my nurses tell the patient when he or she gets the shot," says Ginger Campbell, an ER physician and host of *The Brain Science* podcast. "If patients are given morphine but don't know they got it, the effectiveness of the morphine is decreased. But if they are told they are getting a shot that will ease their pain, they experience relief faster than the morphine can actually take effect. What you tell patients to expect really matters."

Our brains just as eagerly and efficiently prepare us for negative outcomes. Tell a patient he will probably feel nausea, dizziness, or pain after taking a medicine and chances are good that he will experience those exact side effects (this phenomenon is known as nocebo, from the Latin for "I will harm"). We may hope for the best, but we brace ourselves for the worst. So while positive expectations can rev up the neurochemical pathways that can bring relief, negative expectations can trigger those that can make us feel our pain more acutely.

The success of the placebo effect sometimes lies in the fact that humans are trainable animals. Remember that biology lesson about Russian physiologist Ivan Pavlov and how he famously conditioned dogs to salivate at the sound of a bell, once they associated that bell with feeding time? Well, as far as the placebo effect is concerned, we may as well be those impressionable canines.

Inject someone with morphine each day for several days, and then give her a saline solution injection, and her body will respond to that injection as if it actually contains morphine. Even our immune system is susceptible to conditioning. Studies have shown that placebos can mimic the effects of the immunosuppression drugs that lower the rejection rate in organ-transplant patients, as well as relieve cold symptoms and allergic skin reactions.

This type of conditioning is mostly unconscious: We don't have to will our bodies to think of saline as morphine. But we are also quick studies. What would a caveman make of the assortment of pills in our medicine cabinets? Absolutely nothing. But we have come to expect certain types of relief from medicines of particular shapes, sizes, and colors. We also expect a certain expertise and competence when we see high-tech equipment, white lab coats, and diplomas on the wall. Doctors know what they are doing, but it also helps that we *believe* they know what they are doing.

What we don't know

Not all placebo effects are created equal. In fact, a patient may not even experience them the same way each time. This is why one of the current goals of research is to accurately quantify the placebo response. Researchers are also trying to home in on the illnesses that are most receptive to placebos. Parkinson's patients, for example, produce more dopamine (a neurotransmitter in the brain that helps regulate motor function) after they are given a placebo injection they are told will relieve their symptoms. Alzheimer's patients, on the other hand, do not seem to benefit from placebos, probably because their withered neural connections disrupt placebo pathways.

And how long does a placebo effect last, anyway? Researchers can't answer that one for sure either, though studies so far have tracked only short-term results. Nor do we know why some people seem immune to placebos. If, after all, human bodies and brains have evolved to respond to placebos, why don't we all respond the same way? "Natural variability can certainly explain the range in response," says Rutgers University evolutionary biologist Robert Trivers, author of *The Folly of Fools: The Logic of Deceit and Self-Deception in Human Life.* "On average, we are susceptible to placebos; that doesn't mean we all are, and it definitely doesn't mean we all exhibit that trait uniformly," says Trivers. There are likely many factors, including genetic ones, at play here. But the bottom line is that there is no simple way to determine who will respond and who won't.

Being able to accurately measure placebo

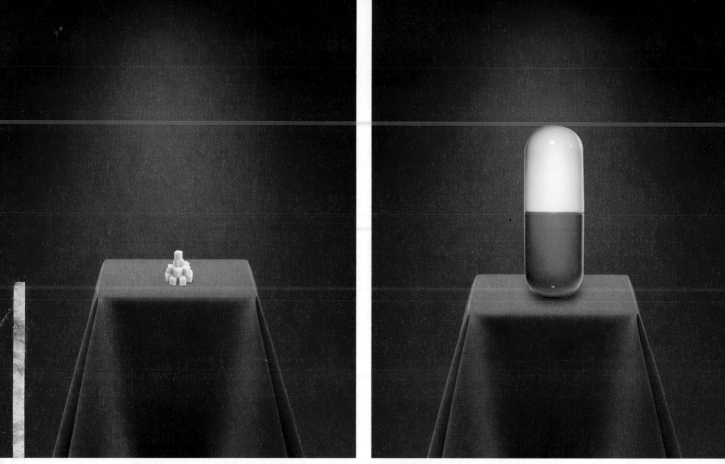

Studies have shown that placebo effects are enhanced by larger and more expensive pills; taking capsules or getting salves and injections has an even more positive effect.

effects is just as important as knowing who will respond. But that, too, is easier said than done. In the 1950s, when researchers first began to use placebos in standardized trials, they knew that participants in the placebo group were likely to improve—healers have always had an intuitive sense of the power of placebos—and that was okay; the group's improvement was the bar the experimental therapy had to clear to be deemed worthy. It is a standard that has served medicine well, and is now, in fact, being used to equal effect to evaluate the latest complementary therapies. But serving passively as the control group in trials is no longer enough. If researchers are going to be able to tap the full potential of placebos, they need to know not only how they stack up against active treatment, but also how they compare with no treatment at all.

In any case, placebo research has a long way to go. And confusing the issue is the fact that every advance comes with some concern. "This is the paradox," says Benedetti. "The more we change the meaning of placebo from negative to positive, the more quacks and shamans feel justified in using new bizarre ways to increase expectations." Yet it's not just the charlatans

who complicate matters. Call it the ethics of deception. Most doctors still believe, and rightly so, that it's just not right to tell a patient he is getting a drug when he isn't. Of course, that patient could be told he is getting "treatment that has been shown to be effective in many cases," and that would be true. But what if patients are told the whole truth? Ted Kaptchuk, who directs placebo studies at Harvard, has demonstrated in clinical trials that placebos can, in fact, work even when patients know they are getting them. It's an intriguing finding, but in the real world of medical care, issues of informed consent are trickier.

For her part, ER physician Campbell wants to make sure one very important lesson isn't lost. "Placebo research highlights the importance of an aspect of medicine that is disappearing: the value of the face-to-face human interaction between the doctor and the patient," she says. Placebos remind us that what matters is not just the active ingredients in a pill. Attention is treatment too.

Who would have thought that the art of healing would one day be supported by the science of placebo effects?

Veronica Skoczek's shared bond with MacGuyver helps treat her symptoms of cerebral palsy.

Doctors With Four Legs

Science has begun to confirm what pet owners have long understood: Sometimes a dog or a cat—or a horse—can provide remarkably effective therapy. **By Beth Howard**

SITTING ASTRIDE HER FAVORITE PONY, MACGUYVER, VERONICA SKOCZEK looks like any other equine-obsessed teenager. With a beaming smile, the pretty 15-year-old expertly maneuvers the brown Connemara-Thoroughbred cross through his paces—walking, trotting, and cantering around the ring. But her easy mastery over the imposing animal contrasts starkly with the lack of control she has over her own body when she is not in the saddle. Skoczek was born with cerebral palsy. Her long limbs contort painfully when she tries to walk. Her torso shudders with spasms.

Before Skoczek began to visit Misty Meadows Mitey Riders, a therapeutic program in Weddington, N.C., her legs tangled with each step; she needed a walker or crutches to get from place to place. "Doctors told her parents that as she got older, she'd need more and more assistance, maybe even a wheelchair to get around," says Erica de Flamand, an instructor with the program. After a year of weekly lessons, Skoczek no

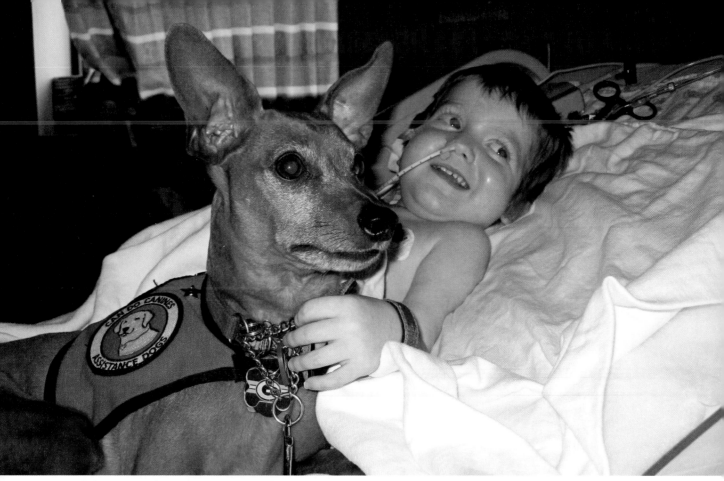

As he recovers from a heart transplant, Saul Hedlund enjoys the company of Dr. Jack, a service dog that sees 15 patients a day at Mayo Clinic's St. Mary's Hospital.

longer needed a walking aid, and her once halting gait had improved dramatically.

Putting kids with disabilities on horseback is just one way the animal kingdom is being employed these days to boost human wellness. Guide dogs, long invaluable sidekicks to the blind, are only the most obvious example. Today service animals are being trained to pull wheelchairs and even detect seizures in companions and call for help. In fact, animal-assisted activities and therapy, like that provided by Misty Meadows Mitey Riders, are a growth industry. Horses, dogs, and cats are being used to ease emotional trauma in war veterans and depression in cancer patients, to calm children facing frightening or painful hospital procedures, and to motivate patients of all ages through the hard grind of rehabilitation.

Shake hands with Dr. Jack

Dr. Jack sees 15 patients over the course of a typical day at Mayo Clinic, integrally involved in the therapy of each. His patients swear by him. Dr. Jack, though, can't check a pulse or write a prescription, because he is a miniature pinscher—an adorable dog, to be sure, but a dog nonetheless. Yet the clinic's resident therapy canine is every inch the professional. "He sees patients on referral from a physician who gives us a set of specific goals they'd like to achieve," explains Marcia Fritzmeier, Dr. Jack's trainer. One of them, Saul Hedlund of Lewiston, Minn., was 3 when, as a complication of a heart transplant, he experienced a loss of muscle control that caused his right fingers to curl up. His therapy included petting Dr. Jack, an action that necessarily required Saul to stretch his fingers. Today the toddler has much more use of his right hand and enjoys leading Dr. Jack around the waiting room when he returns to the hospital for follow-up visits.

Most nonhuman caregivers don't have a job as regular as Dr. Jack's. Pet Partners, an international agency that trains people to be therapy-animal handlers and then pairs them with pets, has 11,000 registered teams in 50 states and 14 other countries. And those 11,000 make over 1 million patient visits each year—to hospitals, nursing homes, physical therapy centers, and other care facilities. There are many more pro-

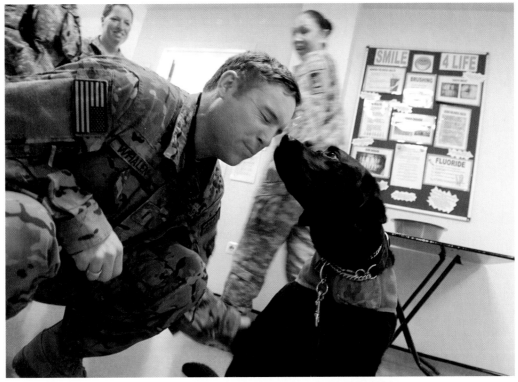

A soldier receives a wet-nosed welcome from a therapy dog at a medical facility in Kandahar, Afghanistan, where canines help patients recover from the traumas of war.

grams just like it. "Our goal is to identify creative ways to engage humans and animals to benefit both ends of the leash," says Rebecca A. Johnson, a registered nurse and the director of the Research Center for Human-Animal Interaction at the University of Missouri at Columbia.

The comfort of contact

The advantages of animal therapy can be intuitively understood by anyone who has ever loved a pet. In fact, virtually any animal—even snakes or lizards in the right hands—can provide "contact comfort," the calming effect of a simple touch. Scientists have found that spending time with a dog or cat (or guinea pig or hamster) lowers blood pressure and respiratory rate, reduces harmful stress hormones like cortisol, and raises the level of oxytocin, a neurochemical produced by breastfeeding mothers that promotes feelings of well-being. Just watching fish swimming in a tank has been shown to reduce blood pressure and anxiety.

That special something we have with our animals dates back thousands of years. In an-

cient Egypt pets were interred or, more often, mummified, an eternal testament to this emotional affinity. The first reported use of animals for therapeutic purposes was in the 18th century. Caring for the rabbits and chickens that roamed the grounds of a British mental hospital helped patients develop better self-control. Sigmund Freud's diaries from the early 20th century reveal that his dog, a chow chow named Jofi, was often by his side during psychoanalysis sessions, putting his patients at ease to share their innermost thoughts.

The modern era of animal-assisted therapy began in the 1960s, with the emergence of data on the healing effects of pet ownership. In a landmark study from the University of Pennsylvania, cardiac patients who had pets were more likely than those who didn't to be alive one year after discharge from the hospital. In fact, only 6% of those pet owners died during that first year, compared with 28% of the petless. Other studies have shown that pet owners are also less likely to need to seek medical care than non-owners, not to mention that people who walk their dogs tend to walk more than those who don't have them,

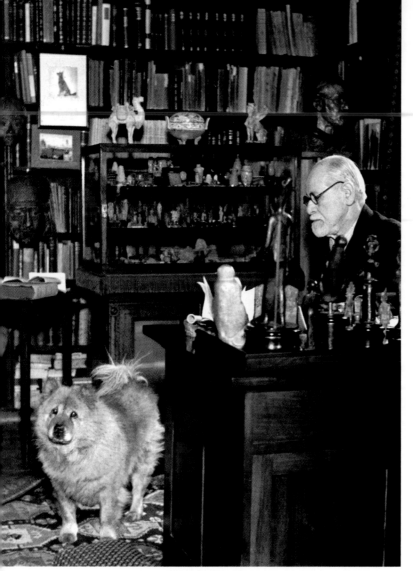

Sigmund Freud's dog Jofi often alerted his master to stress in a patient by choosing where to sit during a session.

calming influences, relaxing patients before nerve-racking procedures like electroconvulsive (shock) therapy or taxing ones like an MRI scan, which requires the patient to stay still in a dark, noisy machine. In essence, these animals are substitutes for commonly prescribed anti-anxiety medications. And unlike those medicines, animals cause no side effects. "Physicians can prescribe animal therapy knowing that they are really prescribing therapy," says Susana Muñoz Lasa, professor of physical and rehabilitation medicine at Complutense University in Madrid.

In the end, dogs and cats are just cuddly, but you can't exactly cuddle a horse, can you? The dynamic between horse and human offers a different way into a patient's psyche. As prey animals, horses are wired to detect danger; they are always assessing possible threats. But that high alertness

and thus are more likely to meet recommended physical activity guidelines.

The evidence keeps piling up. Regular visits from dogs and cats reduced loneliness and depression among residents of a senior living facility. Adding a fish tank to a care ward for Alzheimer's patients, who are often agitated, helped them sit longer—and eat more—at mealtime. And people provided with a canary to look after reported greater psychological well-being after three months than those who were given a plant or nothing at all. "We have a need to nurture, to feel we're responsible for somebody else, and in doing so, we get more of a feeling of control over our world," says Stanley Coren, professor emeritus of psychology at the University of British Columbia at Vancouver and an expert on the power of pets. "Nurturing another gives us a feeling of purpose."

Dogs and cats may do their best work as

also makes them efficient barometers of human feelings of all kinds. "Horses take cues from our body language," says Kris Batchelor, a certified therapeutic riding instructor at Triple Play Farm in Davidson, N.C. "They can even hear our heart beat if we're very close."

And that can give us a window into our own behavior. A victim of abuse who is dealing with feelings of powerlessness, for example, might approach a horse with a particular tentativeness at first. But over time, his ability to exert control over the animal will rebuild his confidence, and the feeling from that experience will then seep into the rest of his life. "As clients begin to build a relationship with the animal, they start to connect the dots," Batchelor says. "In essence, horses are 1,000-pound feedback machines."

That feedback results from doing rather than talking, and because experiences make the strongest impressions, experts say, equine therapy is more likely to produce lasting benefits (say, greater self-esteem in at-risk youth) than conventional therapy. Couples participating in equine-assisted relationship therapy, in which partners both separately and in tandem perform exercises with a horse, are at least as likely to sort out their conflicts as those enrolled in more traditional therapy—in part because a horse senses things a human therapist can't. Small wonder that the U.S. Department of Veterans Affairs has funneled thousands of dollars into programs, such as Horses for Heroes, to help soldiers cope with the psychological fallout of their experiences in Iraq and Afghanistan.

People with debilitating physical conditions—cerebral palsy, multiple sclerosis, muscular dystrophy—people like Veronica Skoczek, rely on a different set of equine assets. Research suggests that the rhythm of a horse's gait mimics the movement of the human pelvis during walking. And this movement seems to stimulate nerves that promote better alignment, muscle symmetry, and postural control among riders. The result, studies show, is a significant improvement in motor function and balance, as well as a lessening of muscle spasticity.

Skoczek has been riding for almost a decade now. Still, each time she takes MacGuyver's reins, the change is obvious. Her tight leg and arm muscles relax, allowing her to execute the careful moves that tell her mount where to go and what to do. "I feel powerful when I am riding," she says. And that power has given her much more control over her own motions.

A couple of years ago, Skoczek took home a blue ribbon in a local horse show. No one but her instructors knew the girl on the big brown horse as anything but a strong, confident rider.

Winning form: Surrounded by her family, Skoczek celebrates after taking first place in a walk/trot equitation event in 2009. "I feel powerful when I am riding," she says.

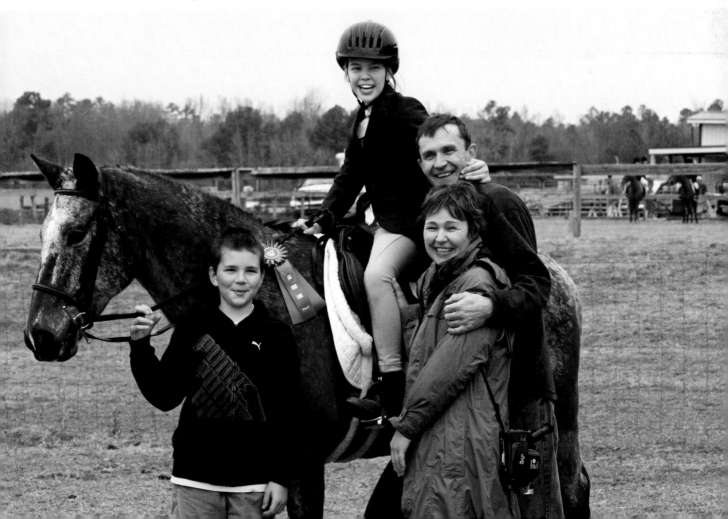

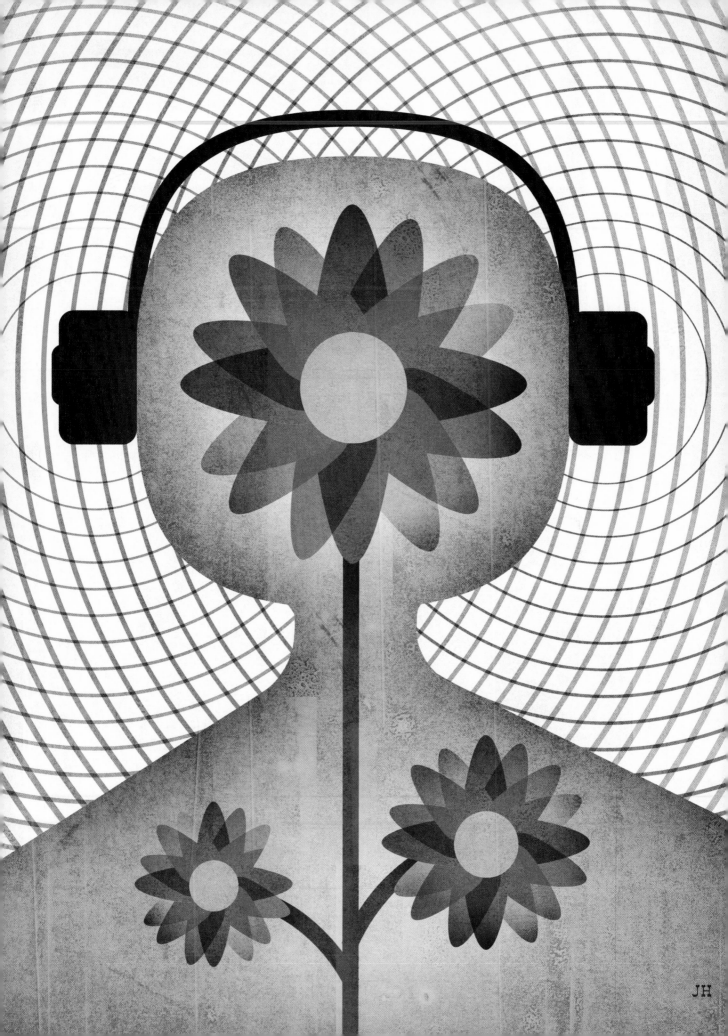

The Sound Of Healing

We all know the power of mood music, but research shows that tuneful therapy is a natural painkiller as well. **By Stacey Colino**

IMAGINE A WORLD WITHOUT MUSIC. IT WOULD BE QUIETER, FOR SURE, BUT IT might also be more painful, maybe even less healthy. Music, put simply, can be good medicine. And not just for the soul. "Certain selections nourish your physical body," says Hal Lingerman, author of *The Healing Energies of Music.* "Others will bring greater health to your mind."

If you've ever relied on a Foo Fighters riff to fire you up for a workout or Handel's *Water Music* to soothe your frayed nerves, you have an idea of what Lingerman is getting at. But those interludes don't begin to hit all the high notes. Music can relieve pain and anxiety, enhance immune function and brain function, alleviate stress, and spur physical rehabilitation. From life's beginning (when it can ease the agony of childbirth and calm babies in neonatal intensive-care units) to its end (comforting those in hospice care and lightening the grief of loved ones), music isn't just the soundtrack of our existence. It can be a conductor of our well-being.

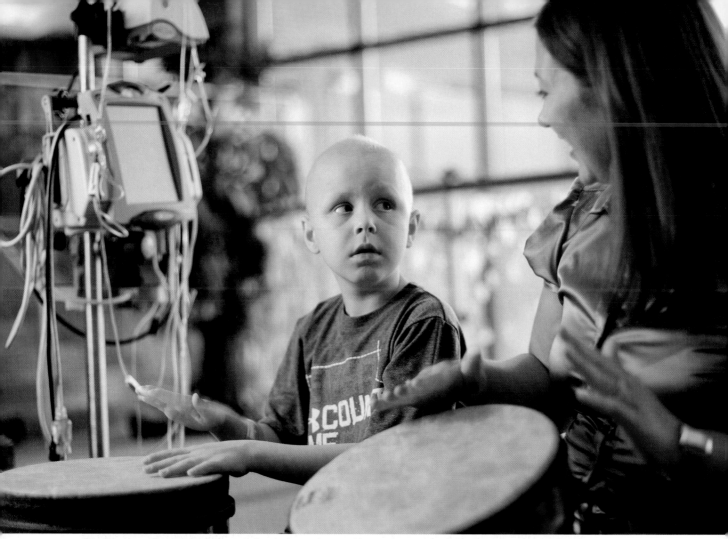

Studies show that music therapy reduces the anxiety and increases the comfort of hospitalized children.

Let's be clear: Music therapy isn't just a fancy way to describe your kicking back with the latest Beyoncé download. It's an evolving and seriously scientific undertaking that has been shown to induce definite changes in central nervous system activity. "Music helps stimulate theta and alpha waves in the brain that are more associated with creativity and insight," explains David Rakel, M.D., director of the University of Wisconsin Integrative Medicine Program. That's right: It can actually help you think more clearly. More important, the right rhythms have been shown to reduce the stress response and increase the relaxation response. And a cooler head can mean a better functioning body.

Okay, so that's not exactly a fresh idea: Aristotle and Plato both wrote about the healing powers of song. But music therapy didn't become a formalized field until after World War II. Musicians often visited veterans' hospitals to entertain those suffering the scars of war, and it didn't take long for doctors and nurses to recognize the posi-

tive effects, both physically and emotionally, that the performances had on patients. Soon facilities were training their own on-premises music makers. Only in the past two decades, though, has the treatment gained a full measure of legitimacy from patients and physicians alike. The reason is simple. "It has a nice intuitive appeal," notes Debra Burns, coordinator of music therapy programs at the Purdue School of Engineering and Technology, "and you'd be hard-pressed to find any documented negative side effects."

Today music therapy is conducted by specially trained practitioners. They choose or produce selections tailored to a patient's tastes and needs, whether the purpose is to ease anxiety before surgery—or distract from pain afterward—or maybe to relieve nausea from chemotherapy or mental and physical tension. No musical style is inherently more therapeutic than others, nor does any one style work for everyone. If you don't like jazz, for example, it's unlikely to provide comforting effects. In some ways, then, music therapy is an art, as therapist and patient collaborate to match the right melodies to the right situation.

Science has clearly confirmed the value of the art. Research in Finland, for instance, found that depressed patients who received music therapy in addition to standard psychotherapy showed better improvement on measures of depression, anxiety, and overall functioning after three months than those who received standard psychotherapy only. And at Mayo Clinic, patients who underwent heart surgery experienced a significant decrease in pain and an easier time relaxing after listening to music that included nature sounds in the days immediately following their procedure. Credit a boost in the levels of oxytocin (often referred to as the love hormone), as another study suggests. In general, when stress levels fall, pain tolerance rises. "The areas of the brain that are related to natural painkillers can be activated by music that has emotional meaning," Burns explains. And that can mean a pharmacological bonus: a decreased need for pain medications.

Music therapy has also been shown to help autistic children, improving their expressive language skills and greasing the wheels of interaction. "Music is a social phenomenon," notes Burns, "so it can teach social skills. When kids with developmental disabilities play music together, they have to attend to what each other is doing." And working together helps them learn to communicate and cooperate better. Similarly, patients with Alzheimer's and other forms of dementia who have lost the ability to speak become more socially engaged when they mouth the words to a familiar song or clap their hands to an engaging rhythm.

Music has also improved the quality of life in people with cancer, lowering levels of anxiety, pain, and depression. Christina Wood, a music therapist at Mayo Clinic, tells of one 50-year-old woman with terminal cancer who was referred to a music therapist by her hospice staff. To ease the woman's pain and nausea and decrease her nighttime restlessness, the therapist combined live and recorded music with deep breathing and guided imagery. Though the patient had been given just a few weeks to live, she survived many months at a higher quality of life. Toward the end, the focus of her therapy shifted to choosing meaningful music for the funeral and pieces that might help loved ones as they grieved.

Most impressively, those who have suffered strokes or brain injuries have regained speech, motor skills, sensory perception, and emotions after undergoing music therapy. After Arizona congresswoman Gabrielle Giffords was shot in the head in January 2011, damaged language pathways in her brain caused her to lose the ability to speak. Music therapy helped train her brain to forge a different route to spoken language. She started by learning to repeat basic phrases in a sing-song voice; as that became easier, she learned short songs that became chants that began to mimic the natural rhythms of speech. Eventually she was uttering phrases to the beat. It's not that much different from learning your ABCs by singing the alphabet song.

The biological phenomenon at the root of some of these improvements is known as entrainment. Simply put, a body's biological rhythms realign with external musical rhythms. So play a slow, soothing tempo for someone who is agitated and his heart rate, blood pressure, and respiratory rate will ease as well. In the same way, music's steady rhythm can improve gait problems in someone who has Parkinson's or who has suffered a brain injury or stroke. "The brain anticipates the space between beats and generates movement accordingly," Wood explains.

It's a finely tuned process, of course, which for best effect should be done under the supervision of a trained professional. But the safety of the therapy, in general, means in many circumstances it can be self-administered as well. "There are so many ways to use music for wellness," Wood says. "The key is to be more intentional about how you listen to it." So the next time you're nervous about a doctor's appointment or an unpleasant procedure, bring along your iPod. Or if you're feeling down, turn up the volume. Sometimes, the only doctor you need is Dr. John.

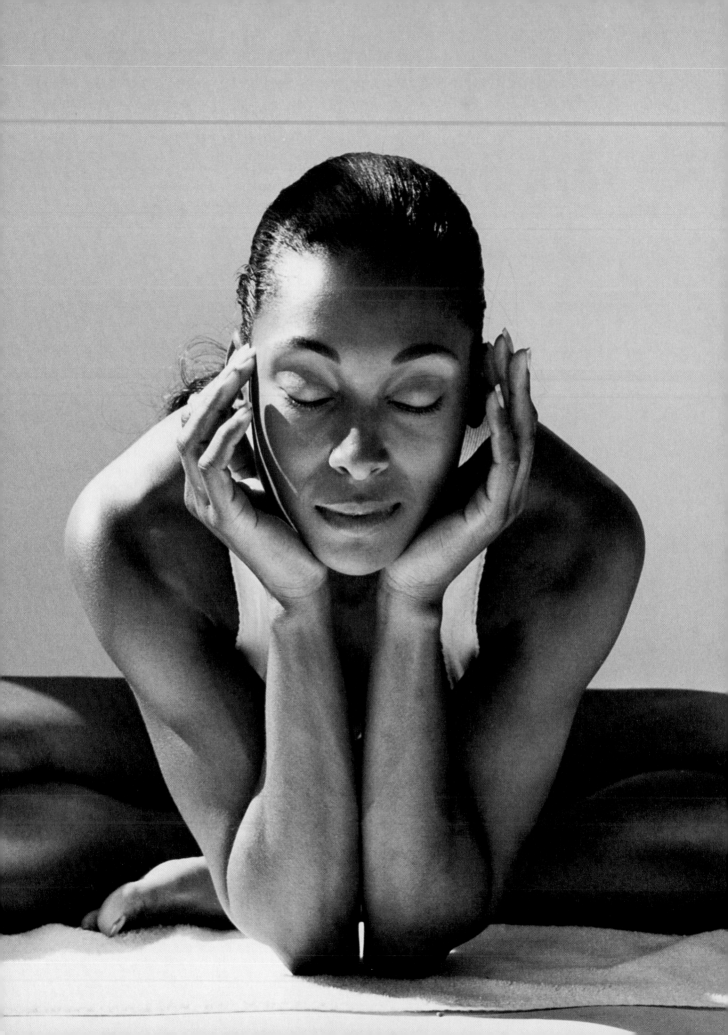

Flexing
And
Calming

Bend and Be Well

Modern medicine is embracing the ancient Indian discipline of yoga, which can help ease ailments ranging from back pain to heart disease. By Lesley Alderman

HARD TO BELIEVE NOW, BUT YOGA WAS ONCE CONSIDERED HERETICAL, even dangerous. As recently as a century ago, yogis in America were viewed with suspicion; some were actually thrown in jail. Today, though, most gyms offer it, many public schools teach it, and a growing number of doctors prescribe it. Yoga studios are as ubiquitous as Starbucks. It may have taken 5,000 years, but yoga has arrived.

Although yoga means "union" in Sanskrit, there are widely diverse ways to practice it. There's gentle yoga and power yoga. Iyengar and Ashtanga. Short classes and long. But almost all offerings share core elements: challenging postures (asanas), focused breathing, self-acceptance. And no multitasking allowed. The poses challenge muscles, while yoga's meditative character calms the mind. All together, yoga activates healthy processes (such as the rest-and-digest response) and deactivates less healthy ones (stress), bringing the body into better balance. Turns out, this ancient Indian prac-

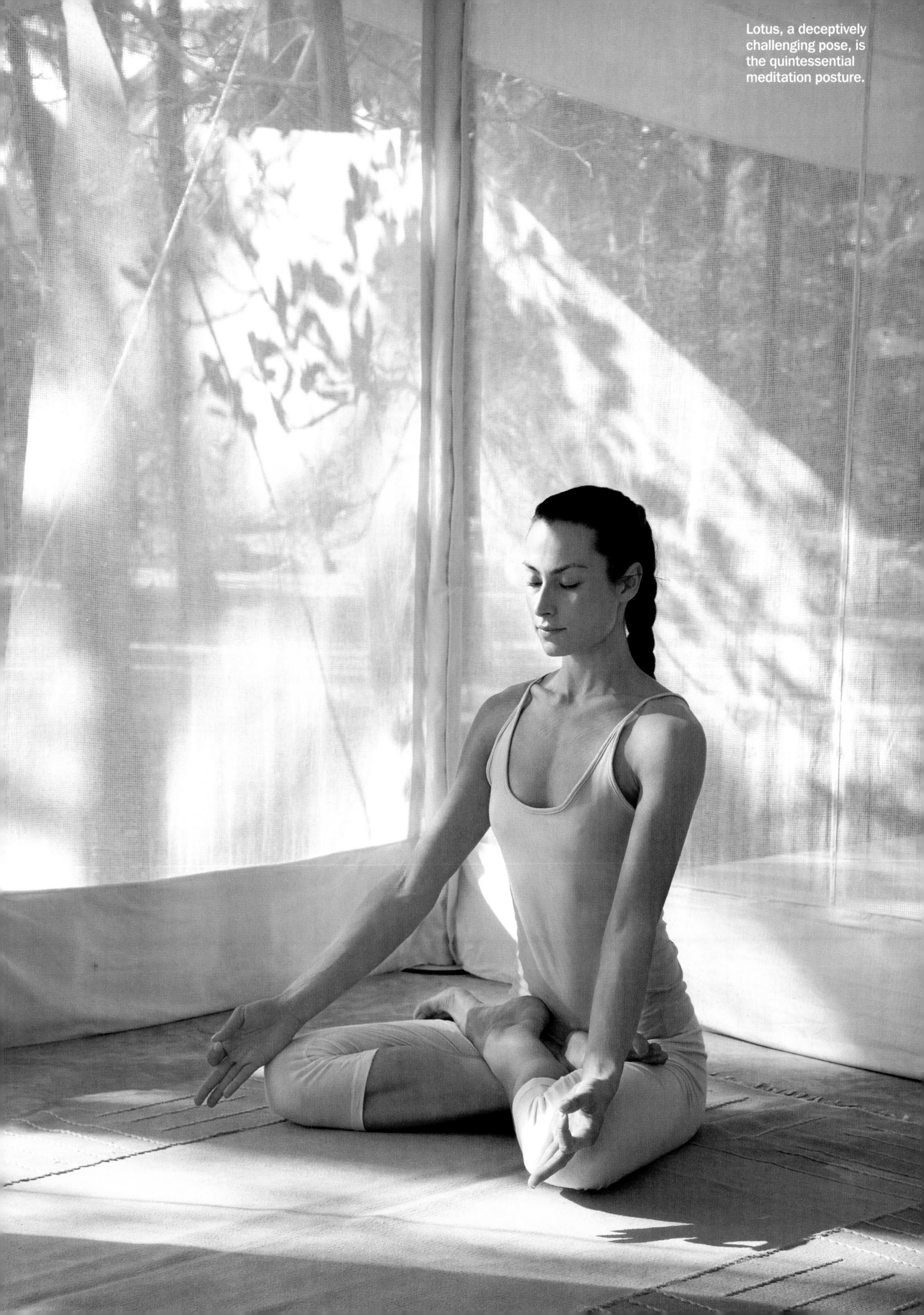

Lotus, a deceptively challenging pose, is the quintessential meditation posture.

WARRIOR II

TREE
POSE

tice is a one-stop antidote to our modern, caffeinated culture. "Yoga is a systematic way to improve the function of everything in the body a little bit," says Timothy McCall, M.D., author of *Yoga as Medicine*. "Keep up the practice, and those improvements tend to deepen over time."

Some of those improvements, a growing body of research suggests, affect an array of particularly hard-to-treat medical problems, including depression, multiple sclerosis, and osteoporosis. And that message is finally getting through. "M.D.s are increasingly comfortable recommending yoga for conditions ranging from lower-back pain to stress," says Baxter Bell, a physician and therapeutic yoga instructor in Oakland, Calif.

As we all know, chronic stress is no joke. Over time it can exacerbate or increase the risk of serious conditions including obesity, heart disease, diabetes, depression, and gastrointestinal problems. "Unfortunately, stress is one condition our culture hasn't found a good way to treat," says Brent Bauer, director of the Mayo Clinic Integrative Medicine Program.

Luckily for our culture, another one has. Researchers at Ohio State University College of Medicine recently compared 25 novice yogis with 25 expert yogis (those who had been practicing at least twice a week for a year or more). The expert yogis had lower blood levels of interleukin-6, a marker of inflammation that often results from stress, which in turn contributes to heart disease and diabetes. In addition, IL-6 levels in the expert yogis increased less after they were subjected to stressors.

Mood disorders also seem to respond positively to yoga. While there are already any number of medicines that boost mood and lower anxiety, too often it is difficult to come up with the right cocktail of drugs for particular patients. And the side effects can be deterring. Yoga, though, has been shown to have a Prozac-like effect on the brain. Researchers at Boston University School of Medicine, for example, monitored two groups of individuals for 12 weeks: One group walked for 60 minutes three times a week, the other spent the same amount of time doing yoga. The yoga group reported lower

levels of anxiety and a greater improvement in mood. As mood rose, so did levels of GABA (gabba-amniobutyric acid), a neurotransmitter that helps promote a state of calm. (Low GABA levels, in contrast, are associated with depression and other anxiety disorders.) "Yoga may work in part by correcting imbalances in the autonomic nervous system caused by stress," says one of the study's authors, Chris Streeter, a Boston University School of Medicine psychiatrist.

A number of small studies have shown that yoga can reduce physical pain too, particularly back pain. One study compared three treatment options over a 12-week period: a weekly yoga class, a weekly stretching class, and reading self-help books on back care. The yoga and stretching groups both improved significantly during and after the trial; these participants had less pain and were able to move more easily than the readers. The study's authors concluded that because the two exercise groups had similar effects, yoga's contribution to alleviating back pain was "largely attributable to the physical benefits of stretching and strengthening the muscles."

And yet the findings, which were published in *Archives of Internal Medicine*, may not tell the whole story. "All the yoga subjects did the exact same moves," notes Loren Fishman, medical director of Manhattan Physical Medicine and Rehabilitation in New York. "In real life, patients with back pain would be given a series of poses tailored to their diagnosis. Someone with a herniated disc would be treated very differently from someone with spinal stenosis. So the results could be even better."

Fishman brings up an interesting point. The many different versions of yoga provide an opportunity to customize therapy. So to optimize yoga's benefits, patients should first consult a doctor to help pinpoint a class or style for their specific ail-

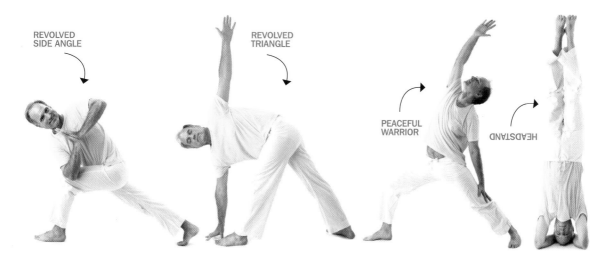

REVOLVED SIDE ANGLE

REVOLVED TRIANGLE

PEACEFUL WARRIOR

HEADSTAND

ment. While a general yoga class may help with problems like stress and depression, particular problems like arthritis may well require a more specialized class or customized routine.

In any case, most yoga will help keep the heart healthy by reducing stress levels and blood pressure. A study conducted at the University of Pennsylvania found that after participating in a three-month yoga course, participants with hypertension or pre-hypertension had significantly lower blood pressure. And a review of more than 70 studies by the Center for the Study of Complementary and Alternative Therapies at the University of Virginia found that yoga may be instrumental in improving glucose tolerance and insulin sensitivity, cholesterol and triglyceride profiles, and blood pressure, all factors that contribute to cardiovascular problems. What's more, yoga encourages heart rate variability, which, perhaps counterintuitively, reduces heart disease risk.

And while you are building heart health, you may be building bone strength as well. A 2009 study by Fishman found that just 10 minutes of yoga a day helped build bone mineral density in middle-aged subjects. How does yoga build bone? Simply, bending and twisting stimulate osteocytes, the cells that make bone. Because yoga isn't a traditional weight-bearing workout, however, it shouldn't damage cartilage or lead to osteoarthritis, both common consequences of strength training.

Speaking of joint pain, rheumatoid arthritis is an autoimmune disease that causes painful inflammation of joints and surrounding tissues. Conventional treatments, including steroids, can have serious and unpleasant side effects such as heart problems and weight gain. Once again, preliminary research shows yoga may be an appropriate alternative. An Indian study found that participants of a one-week yoga camp who practiced breathing exercises and yoga poses twice a day lowered their stress and anxiety levels and were able to perform basic tasks, including dressing and eating, more easily. What's more, the subjects' rheumatoid factor levels, the most relevant marker of the disease, dropped. It was not clear why yoga helped reduce those levels, but the study's lead author, Shirley Telles, head of the Indian Council of Medical Research Center for Advanced Research in Yoga and Neurophysiology at Bangalore, theorizes that the carefully designed yoga program helped "correct the imbalance in the immune system."

Finally, a Mayo study found significant positive effects on its own employees after just six weeks of a yoga-based wellness program that included nutritional counseling and meditation. In particular, the participants displayed reductions in blood pressure and stress, and an increase in flexibility. What was especially encouraging to the researchers was that the participants attended class six days a week at 5:10 a.m. in the dead of winter, and yet, according to Mayo's Brent Bauer, "We had to turn people away in droves." That, more than anything else, he says, speaks to the interest that yoga is generating as people get increasingly concerned about contributing to their own wellness.

They're making a good call. Yoga's reach seems to extend to most corners of the body, from the nervous system to the circulatory system to the immune system. But in the end, most of yoga's advantages are a result of its overall calming influence. "Yoga is about learning to be where you are in this moment and not trying to be somewhere else or in some other body," says Barbara Verrochi, co-director of the Shala Yoga House, a New York studio. After a few months of yoga, there may be no other body you'd rather be in.

It Hurts
So Good

Millions of patients are dragging chiropractic and massage therapies into mainstream medicine—for good reason. Their satisfaction and reams of data show it works. By Bryan Walsh

I'M LYING ON MY STOMACH, HEAD WEDGED INTO A CUSHIONED FACE REST that leaves just enough space for me to breathe. The position itself should be sufficient to generate no small amount of apprehension, but there's also this: I'm naked, save for the sheet draped over my posterior. Yet I'm as relaxed as I've ever been, the tension in my body—and especially that knot I've felt in my right side for years—dissolving in waves. I can even forgive the chanting that's playing quietly in the background. All thanks to the massage therapist standing over me, her fingers kneading the small of my back, arranging and rearranging my muscles until I feel as soft and pliable as Silly Putty. At the moment, I don't particularly care about the medical benefits of massage. All I need to know is that it feels good.

I have joined the blissful state shared by a growing number of patients taking advantage of what has come to be known as "manipulative medicine." According to the National Institutes of Health, an estimated 18 million adults in the U.S. receive

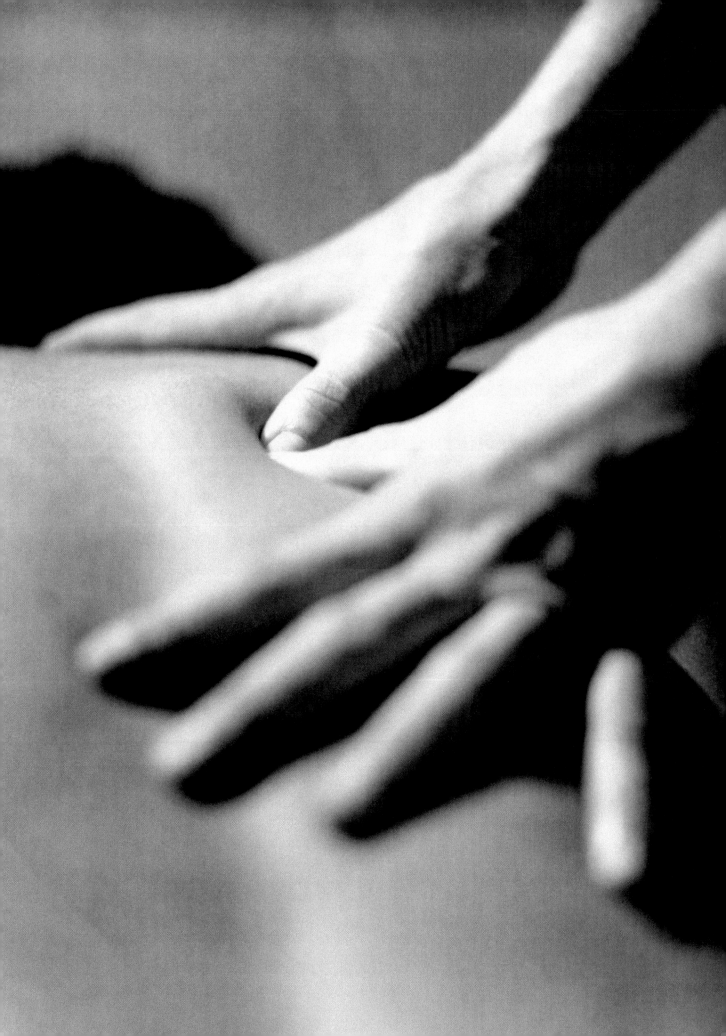

Chiropractors treat more than 30 million patients annually. Doctors have only recently begun to understand the physiology of manipulative medicine.

massage therapy each year. Chiropractors—those back-cracking spinal manipulators—treat more than 30 million of us annually. Those are robust numbers for a pair of alternative practices that once were barely considered legitimate by the medical establishment. Decades ago the American Medical Association branded chiropractic an "unscientific cult," and massage therapy still has to contend with a slightly seamy backroom reputation. (Hey, what happened on *The Client List* this week?) But these days, manipulative medicine is pretty much mainstream. According to a 2011 survey by Health Forum and Samueli Institute, more than 42% of responding hospitals indicated they offer one or more complementary and alternative-medicine therapies, up from 37% in 2007. Massage therapy was one of the top two services provided.

But even patients who swear by their massage therapist or chiropractor do so less because they know exactly why their visits make them feel better than because they simply do. They're in good company. The fact is, doctors have only recently begun to understand the physiology of manipulative medicine.

For starters, studies have shown that massage therapy, which takes many forms but almost always involves rubbing, pressing, or otherwise manipulating the soft tissues of the body, can increase the body's output of endorphins and serotonin, chemicals that act as natural pain-killers and mood regulators. At the same time, massage also reduces levels of cortisol, a stress hormone. Research published in the *Journal of Alternative and Complementary Medicine* suggests one explanation for this effect: Scientists at Cedars-Sinai Hospital in Los Angeles found that a single deep-tissue Swedish massage led to a more significant decrease in arginine vasopressin (AVP) hormone than a control treatment of light-touch therapy. AVP constricts blood vessels and increases blood pressure, both of which are markers of stress.

Another study, published in the journal *Science Translational Medicine,* showed that massage turns off genes associated with inflammation and the pain that results from it. That, in turn, helps relieve the muscle soreness that follows physical activity or injury. Stack this anti-pain effect on top of the anti-anxiety benefits and you can see why many hospitals—including Mayo Clinic—have begun to incorporate massage therapy into post-surgical treatment.

Still, the studies are only confirming what most of us already know. Pain relief? Relaxation? No kidding. The benefits of massage really do go beyond the most obvious ones. Research by Tiffany Field, director of the Touch Research Institute at the University of Miami School of Medicine, shows that moderate- to deep-pressure massage can activate the vagus nerve, which helps regulate heartbeat. Field also found that massage can help with everything from relief from depression to weight gain in premature infants, and she suspects that an energized vagus nerve may explain why.

Massage offers the kind of benefits that cancer patients can appreciate as well. A 2007 study published in the *Journal of Integrative Oncology* found that after learning massage techniques in short workshops, partners of cancer patients were able to give treatments that reduced anxiety, pain, nausea, and other side effects of cancer by up to 44%. As is often the case with complementary treatments, the researchers hypothesized that it wasn't so much the therapy itself—after all, the massages weren't even given by professionals—as it was the intimacy of the contact that conferred the positive result. On the other hand, that AVP study mentioned above found that massage seemed to raise the production of the cancer-fighting white blood cells known as lymphocytes, and that is much less likely to be a result of such a placebo effect.

Neither cancer nor post-op healing is the primary battleground of massage. The condition that drives more patients to massage therapists and chiropractors than any other is much more mundane: back pain. According to the American Chiropractic Association, more than 30 million Americans suffer from back pain at any given time, and if you're not among them at the moment, chances are you will be eventually. An estimated 80% of us will fall prey sooner or later.

And when you're hurting, fast relief is all that's on your mind. Research indicates that spinal manipulation—a chiropractor's application of force at specific joints of the spine (hence the cracking that chiropractic sessions are known for)—is a good place to start. A 2010 study published in the *Annals of Internal Medicine* showed that chiropractic treatment of neck pain pro-

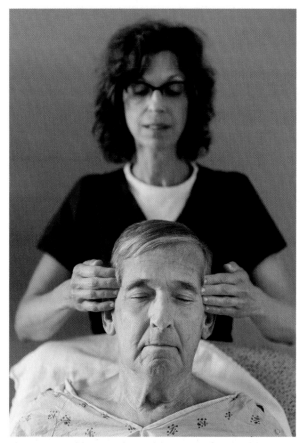

Massage can increase the body's output of endorphins and serotonin, chemicals that act as natural painkillers and mood regulators.

vided more relief than over-the-counter drugs like aspirin and ibuprofen. Specifically, after 12 weeks of treatment, more than half of chiropractic subjects reported at least a 75% reduction in pain, compared with one-third of those in the drug group.

The improvement seemed to last; a year later, more than 50% of the chiropractic group still reported a significant decrease in pain. Meanwhile,

those patients taking painkillers tended to have upped their dosage by the time of the follow-up, and that meant an added bonus for the members of the chiropractic group: They didn't have to worry about the side effects the drug group was contending with.

Which isn't to imply that chiropractic treatment is without controversy. Years ago neurologists noticed a pattern of people suffering strokes following chiropractic adjustment for neck pain. Many implicated the sudden neck twisting that is central to the treatment, hypothesizing that it injured the arteries leading to the brain, thus triggering strokes. But more recent research is causing doctors to rethink that assumption. A 2010 study found that younger stroke patients were more likely to have complained about head and neck pain—symptoms that often precede a stroke—before their visit to the chiropractor, and that could mean they were already suffering the effects of damaged arteries before they underwent any manipulations.

If that's the case, the only significant risk of manipulative medicine may be to your wallet. Just 3% or so of Americans who got a massage over the past five years were covered by health insurance for the treatment, according to a 2010 survey by the American Massage Therapy Association. Massage therapists aren't considered licensed medical practitioners, which means their work isn't recognized by most insurers. On the other hand, almost 90% of insured Americans are covered for chiropractic treatment, because licensed chiropractors, like physicians, have undergone four years of schooling.

For now, there is still no national standard for massage therapists, making it that much more important to scout out a therapist you can trust. Then again, anyone who is prepared to lie face down, naked, on an odd table, in a room with a stranger, probably has done that due diligence already.

Kneads Test

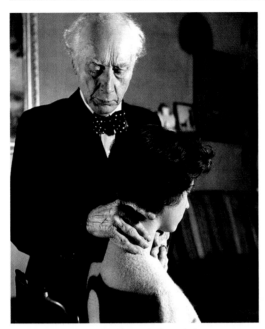

Studies show that F.M. Alexander's technique may enhance respiratory function in adults. Reflexology treatment (below) relieves symptoms of multiple sclerosis.

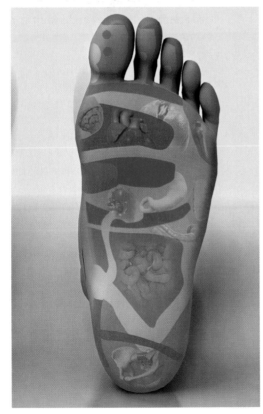

Move beyond the popular and straightforward kneadings of Swedish or shiatsu massage, and most versions of hands-on therapy continue to fall more under the heading of "if it feels good, do it" than "because it does good, do it." Here are some that it won't hurt to try, even if in most cases there is only limited evidence that they offer measurable relief.

Alexander technique: Named for the Australian-English actor, F.M. Alexander, who developed it, this method focuses on the link between the body's posture and movements and its physical problems. Stand or move differently, the thinking goes, and you can relieve or prevent injury. Though little research has been conducted on the Alexander technique, many doctors believe it is worth a try for anyone looking to relieve chronic pain.

Feldenkrais method: Think yoga, minus the obsession with specific positioning. This technique aims for dexterous and painless body movement, with the goal of building better body awareness. That makes it similar to the Alexander technique. Another thing in common? Limited research on its effectiveness.

Rolfing: This deep-tissue massage was developed by the biochemist Ida Rolf, who discovered that the connective tissue surrounding muscles thickens and stiffens with age. Rolfing practitioners use fingers, knuckles, even knees, to knead that tissue in an effort to loosen it up, improving posture and realigning the body. Some people find Rolfing helpful, but be warned: It can be painful, and certain conditions—advanced osteoporosis, for example—can be made worse by the therapy.

Reflexology: Popular throughout Asia, reflexology works off the assumption that specific spots on the soles of the feet correspond to various other parts of the body. Massage the foot in a certain place and relieve pressure or tension in the neck, or even the liver. Reflexology can't harm you, and many people find it relaxing, but there's scant evidence of the purported foot-body pathways.

Spinal manipulation: Lots of studies have shown that spinal manipulation can treat mild to moderate back pain, and some other conditions like headache as well. But some chiropractors also believe they can heal many other conditions and diseases by properly aligning the skeleton; there isn't much research to back up those claims. There are some risks, especially for those who suffer from osteoporosis or nerve damage.

The Mystery Of Acupuncture

Why it works is a matter of debate, but research shows that the ancient technique is effective for treating everything from menopause to backaches. By Jeffrey Kluger

THE HISTORY OF MEDICINE IS THE HISTORY OF PREPOSTEROUS IDEAS that turned out to be right. Illness couldn't be caused by invisible creatures that invade the body. Then Antonie van Leeuwenhoek invented the microscope and we discovered bacteria. Deliberately infecting people with an extremely mild case of a disease shouldn't be the best way to protect them from catching a serious case of it. Then Edward Jenner hit upon smallpox immunization and the era of the vaccine was born.

And you shouldn't be able to treat all manner of afflictions from headaches to backaches to depression to addiction by letting someone stick needles into any number of 360 specific spots on your skin. Especially if the best explanation anyone can give you for why the treatment works is that it frees up the life force, or "qi," that flows though the human body along 14 different lines, or "meridians."

Yet the lure (some would say lore) of the ancient Chinese art of acupuncture is

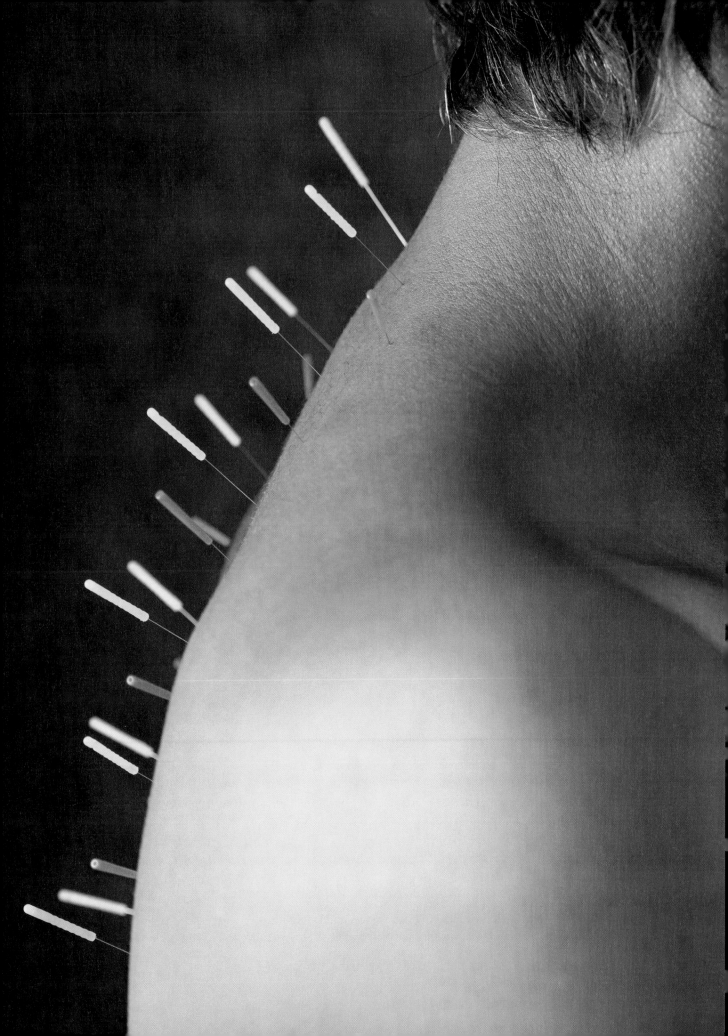

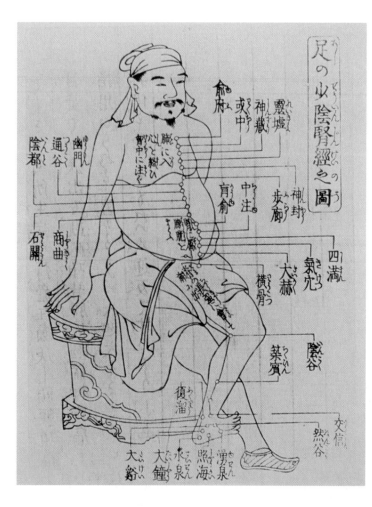

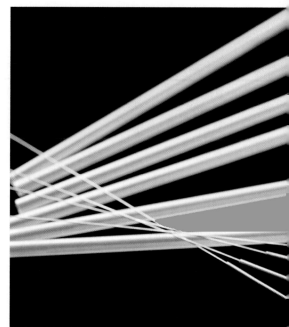

From left: An illustration from China showing acupuncture points on the human body; the thin, solid needles used in the practice; and Lance Corporal Tristin Bell of Billings, Mont., receiving acupuncture in Afghanistan to relieve headaches suffered in the aftermath of an injury.

irresistible all the same, and not only in the Far East. The World Health Organization has declared acupuncture a useful adjunct for more than 50 medical conditions, including emotional woes like chronic stress. In the U.S., the National Institutes of Health (NIH) agrees, endorsing acupuncture as a potentially useful treatment for addiction, migraines, menstrual cramps, abdominal pain, tennis elbow, nausea resulting from chemotherapy and more. NIH statistics from 2007 showed that 3.1 million American adults and 150,000 children had undergone acupuncture in the previous year. From 2002 to 2007, the number of adult users alone jumped by more than 1 million.

In 2009, the U.S. Air Force became a believer too, implementing battlefield acupuncture in Iraq and Afghanistan—a treatment that can include the implantation of semipermanent needles in key acupoints to block or disrupt pain signals. Acupuncture is increasingly used by the military to deal with post-traumatic stress disorder as well. Now NATO forces are considering following the Americans' lead. The Chinese military, of course, uses it routinely.

Civilian practitioners have embraced acupuncture in an even bigger way. Leading American hospitals like Mayo Clinic and the Cleveland Clinic offer it as part of their alternative-care packages. And numerous groups—including the American Medical Association—are pushing to get either the federal government or the states to designate acupuncture an "essential health benefit" under the 2010 Affordable Care Act. The move would require health insurers to include it on their list of covered services.

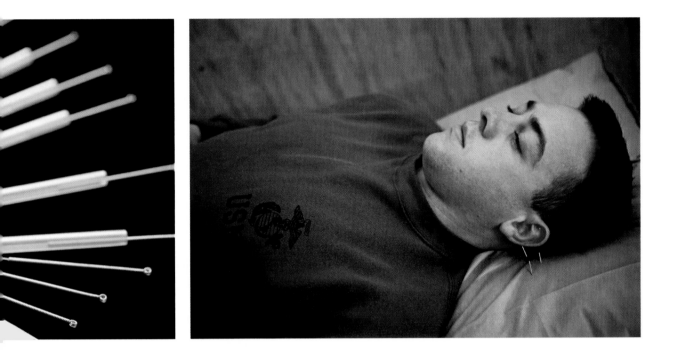

But just because a treatment is popular—even one that has been around for millennia—doesn't guarantee that it is effective. If it were, we'd long since have cleansed, Rolfed, and low-carbed our way to immortality. More and more, though, acupuncture is getting the close empirical scrutiny that modern drugs and medical procedures are routinely subjected to. And the results are, well, mixed.

A growing body of experimental evidence shows that acupuncture does indeed work—in some cases extraordinarily well. Another body suggests that it may very well work, but not for the reasons believers think. And yet a third body of "beats me" findings is sufficient to keep partisans on both sides arguing. In any case, something is clearly going on—and that something may, at least in some cases, be a cure for what ails you.

Crunching the numbers

After colds and flu, pain is the most common cause of visits to physicians—with lower-back pain clocking in at No. 1 on that very long list. Up to 85% of us will eventually suffer from back pain of some kind. Untreated—or inadequately treated—

it's the most common reason for disability claims and employee absenteeism.

Acupuncture is often recommended as one way to treat the problem. In 2007 investigators at the University of Regensburg in Germany gathered a group of 1,162 patients with long histories of lower-back pain to determine whether it could actually make a difference.

Patients were given two half-hour treatment sessions per week for five weeks. About a third of the group underwent traditional, lower-back acupuncture, with needles inserted at the prescribed points. Another third got sham acupuncture, which involved real needles inserted at random spots on the lower back. The remaining third received conventional treatment, consisting of physical therapy and exercise, along with the drugs they were taking.

At the end of the five weeks, the subjects were examined to determine how much pain relief they'd gotten and to what extent their physical functioning had improved. The results: 47.6% of the real acupuncture group experienced significant relief in both categories; in the sham acupuncture group, 44.2% did. In the traditional group, it was just 27.4%. The researchers saw the glass as more than half full, writing sunnily that "acupuncture gives physicians a promising and effective treatment option for lower-back pain, with few adverse effects or contra-indications."

But does it? There is no denying that both groups that received some kind of acupuncture did better than the one that didn't. But there's also no denying that the results of the sham procedure make the idea of 360 carefully mapped entry points on the body look a little silly. Problem is, results like that aren't at all uncommon in acupuncture research—and that's not the best news for a treatment trying to prove its worth.

In 2011, for example, a study at Sweden's Karolinska Institute separated patients suffering from chemotherapy-related pain and nausea into the same three experimental groups: real acupuncture, sham acupuncture, and conventional therapy. This time the sham acupuncture involved blunt needles that didn't even break the skin. Again, both the fake and real groups showed improvement—both more than the Western medicine group. In yet another study, this one looking at the effects of acupuncture on women trying to get pregnant through in vitro fertilization, sham acupuncture actually produced better results—a higher pregnancy rate—than the real thing.

"When a treatment is truly effective, studies tend to produce more convincing results as time passes and the weight of evidence accumulates," wrote Harriet Hall, a former Air Force flight surgeon and an alternative-medicine skeptic, in a 2011 issue of the *Journal of Pain*. "Taken as a whole, the published (and scientifically rigorous) evidence leads to the conclusion that acupuncture is no more effective than a placebo."

Critics also point out that despite the common wisdom that even if acupuncture doesn't help, it can't hurt, there are, in fact, risks involved. Pregnant women, people with a bleeding disorder, and people with a pacemaker (because of possible interference from the mild electricity that is sometimes applied to the needles) should be especially cautious. Even healthy people can suffer organ injury, infection, or soreness if the procedure isn't performed well.

And yet for every study that yields murky or even negative results, plenty of others present a clear win for the pro-acupuncture camp. Women going through menopause received significant relief for their hot flashes and mood swings with acupuncture, and those who got real acupuncture showed far more improvement than those who got the sham version. What's more, blood tests bolstered the results, showing that the level of estrogen rose while luteinizing hormone fell significantly after real acupuncture—the opposite of the direction those hormones usually move during menopause.

Similarly, the U.S. National Institute on Drug Abuse found that real acupuncture—with needles inserted in spots in the ear said to modulate cravings—is overwhelmingly more effective than the fake kind or none at all in treating cocaine addiction. In patients who underwent the proper needle sticks, 53.8% had clean drug screens at the end of the study, compared with 23.5% of subjects getting the sham routine and 9.1% of those who received no acupuncture at all.

Whatever the exact numbers, some relief is obviously better than none—even if it's sometimes conferred by what seems to be the power of the placebo. Besides, it's an enduring truth of the placebo effect that in order for a patient to experience relief, something has to have changed in the body.

So when it comes to acupuncture—real or fake—what is that something?

How it works

Functional magnetic resonance imaging (fMRI) has revealed that when volunteers are subjected to mild electrical shock while undergoing acupuncture, there is much less activity in four different pain-processing regions of the brain than usual. Although the pain stimulus continues, the brain notices it less. A fifth region—the anterior insula, which governs the expectation of pain—quiets down too. Often, the less pain you expect to feel, the less you do feel—a tail-wagging-the-dog phenomenon that is key to the placebo effect. If sham acupuncture produces only partial results, it may be because it affects only the insula rather than all the areas that deal with pain sensation. In any case, something happens. "Acupuncture is supposed to act through at least two mechanisms: nonspecific expectancy-based effects and specific modulation of the incoming pain signal," says Nina Theysohn of University Hospital in Essen, Germany, who conducted the MRI study.

Naturally occurring brain opiates appear to be activated by acupuncture as well: Imaging studies show that mu-opioid receptors—the molecular attachment sites that help nerve cells process the pain-relieving chemicals—have improved binding ability after treatment. Brain scans have also helped to validate an important part of the acupuncturist's art: the rotation of the needles that leads to something known as "de qi," in which the body's tissue seems to grab hold of the metal. There's nothing mysterious about this; tissue fibers actually wind around the needle, making it significantly more difficult to remove it. Patients may report a tingle or electric sensation when de qi occurs, and this too travels to the brain, quieting pain centers. The tradeoff is a slug of analgesic effect for a little pinprick.

Ultimately, it's this minimally invasive quality that makes acupuncture so appealing. Yes, a natural skittishness accompanies being punctured by needles—even exceedingly fine ones. And yes, those punctures can hurt a bit, depending on where the needles are inserted, and how deftly. But once they're in place, treatment requires nothing more than that you lie still and relax.

Maybe acupuncture produces enduring results, maybe it doesn't. But as with any complementary treatment, it's meant to be taken as part of a buffet of choices. And when you are suffering from something as frustrating as chronic pain, why wouldn't you try whatever might help?

"It's the effects of the treatment that are important to the patient, even if those effects are caused by unspecific factors," says the Karolinska Institute's Anna Enblom, who conducted one of the sham-acupuncture studies. Sure, we need to figure out what those factors are, but that's a job for doctors and other scientists. The patients' only job is to reap the rewards.

Pinpoint Accuracy

Research hasn't yet verified what acupuncture can do, so we asked Mark C. Lee, Mayo Clinic's physician acupuncturist, to rate (on a five-point scale) the therapy's apparent helpfulness in five major areas.

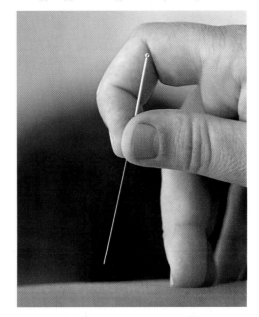

Pain management
(5 for helpfulness; 5 for evidence)
Many studies have found success in easing back, neck, and arthritis pain, as well as migraines, menstrual cramps, and the discomfort of carpal tunnel syndrome.

Mental health
(4 for helpfulness; 3 for evidence)
Most evidence shows a fair amount of promise in lessening anxiety, stress, and insomnia, but not as much for depression.

Addiction
(3 for helpfulness; 3 for evidence)
Auricular acupuncture, placing needles in the outer ear, is useful in treating dependency on cigarettes, alcohol, and other drugs.

Gastrointestinal disorders
(5 for helpfulness; 4 for evidence)
Growing evidence demonstrates benefits in managing nausea and constipation.

Respiratory disorders
(2 for helpfulness; 1 for evidence)
There are some indications that sinusitis, sore throat, hay fever, and the common cold may respond to treatment.

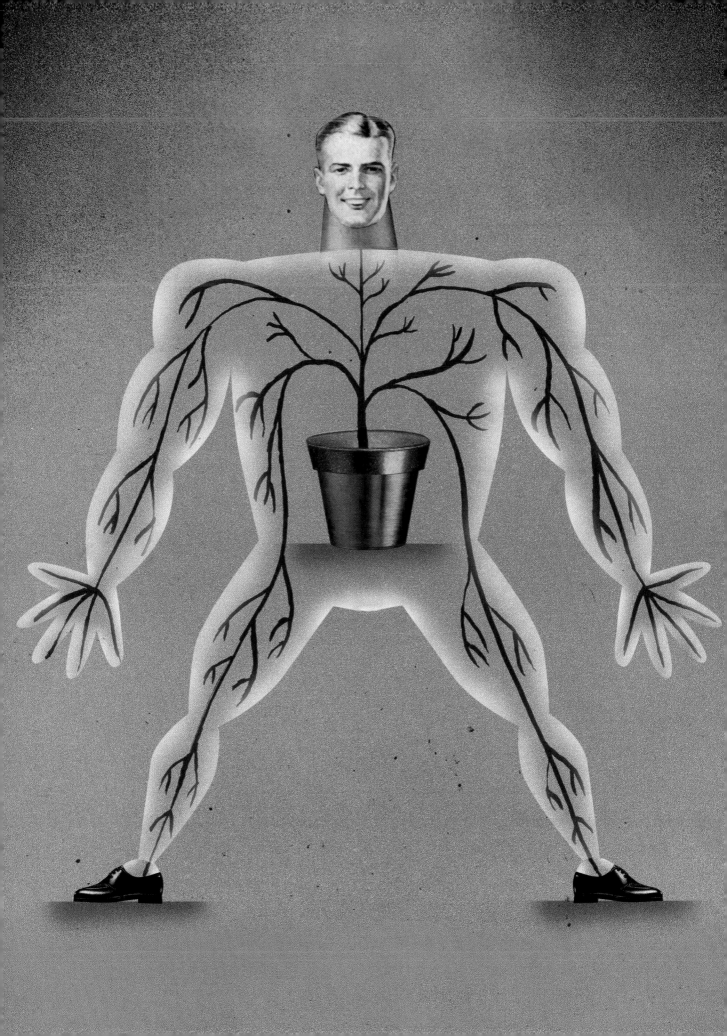

Healing
Naturally

Pain, Pain, Go Away

When the hurt lingers, the physical discomfort is only part of the problem. Easing the emotional toll may offer the most relief.
By Lori Oliwenstein

PAIN IS A SYMPTOM, NOT A DISEASE. THE MEDICAL TEXTS SAY SO. SO DID your mom ("It's only a bruise! Stop acting like you're dying!"). But while most of us knee-bangers, finger-cutters, and bone-breakers know that pain is just the body alerting us to a pathological process going on inside us, it is such an in-your-face message that it never fails to attract our attention. Make that *grab* our attention.

That is, after all, much of what pain is about: attention. Hey you, over here! And if you can feel it and isolate it, you can manipulate it—obliterate the source, maybe, but at least mitigate the factors that pump up its volume or redirect your focus from the throbbing. Because while pain is about attention and sensation, it is also about emotion. That emotional component, of course, has been a boon, evolutionarily speaking; since the Stone Age, survival has often depended on finding pain compelling enough to do whatever is needed to make it—and whatever is causing it—go away.

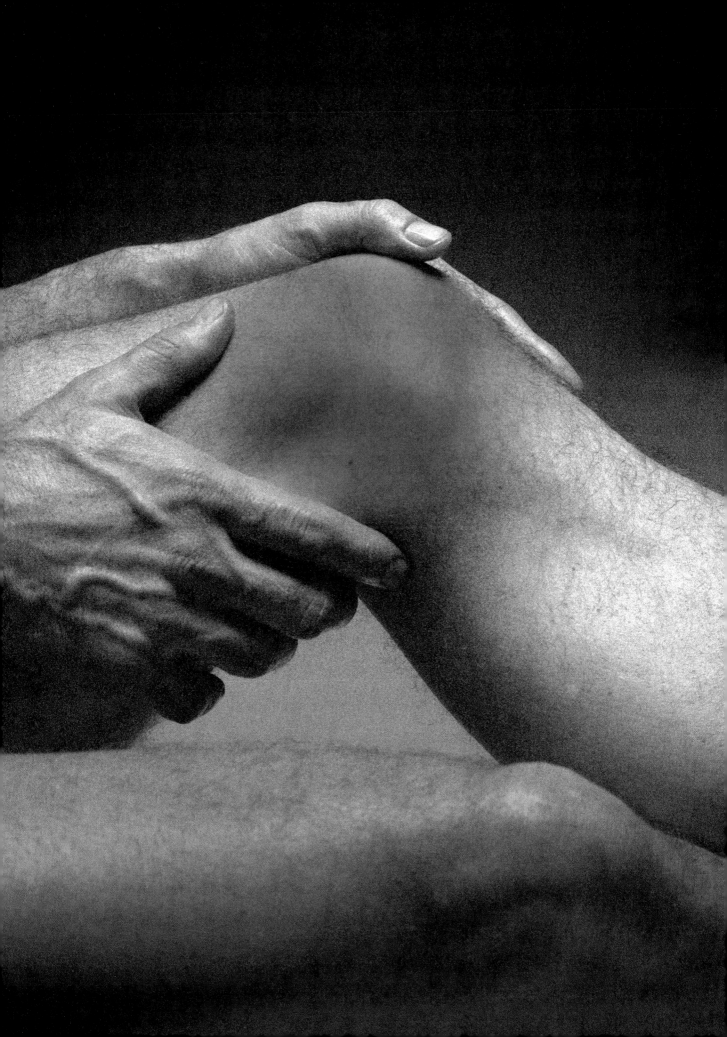

Attention, sensation, emotion. Those factors, says W. Michael Hooten, a pain specialist and associate professor of anesthesiology at Mayo Clinic, are the foundation of a kind of web in the brain. This web connects the parts that detect pain signals with those that respond to the signals emotionally via chemical messengers called neurotransmitters. Break some of the web's threads and distract those messengers, and you can free yourself from its clutches. Maybe the underlying pathology will still be there, but it will no longer be a pain in your ... whatever.

Scientists call it the pain matrix, and here's how it works: You bend over to pick up a carton of books but forget the old advice to lift with your legs. Before you've fully straightened up, you detect trouble. Part of that realization comes from the actual sensation, recognized instantly by your suddenly hyperactive somatosensory cortex, the piece of the brain that receives and interprets the signals now racing up your spine.

Chances are, though, that when you felt that first twinge, you regarded it with something other than clinical calm. Your breath caught in your throat. You cursed or yowled. Maybe you cried. In short, you responded emotionally. Acute pain knows how to get your attention and elicit strong feelings, emotional and physical.

Brain-imaging studies can actually show us what this looks like. "With a pain signal, we see activation in the prefrontal cortex and anterior cingulate cortex, two areas of the brain that are important to providing emotional color to the pain experience," Hooten explains. "Focusing on the pain drives up activity in these emotional centers."

Normally, the three components of the pain matrix are in balance. Stub your toe and you hop up and down in pain, screaming in anger. But within minutes, if not seconds, the throbbing begins to subside, and with it, your emotions ebb too.

Sometimes, however, the pain doesn't go away. Faced with an unceasing barrage of pain signals, the brain falls a bit out of sync. Because it can only surmise that its neurochemical distress calls are going unheeded, it yells louder. And

louder. At some point, the emotional component of the pain becomes the predominant signal, and feeding on itself, it can end up lasting long after the actual pain stimulus is gone or reduced.

Chronic pain, by definition, is hard to solve. And when conventional medicine falls short, complementary therapies often get the call. You're not likely to run to an acupuncturist or massage therapist for that stubbed toe, but for a migraine that won't quit? Anything to silence the roar.

At their core, most integrative pain-reducing techniques try to get the brain to shift attention, to decrease the chemicals, like cortisol, that make you feel stressed, while increasing those—serotonin, say, or norepinephrine—that make you feel happy or calm.

Take acupuncture. It has been shown to reduce the severity of sensation in everything from back pain to migraines, post-surgical pain to battlefield traumas. The traditional explanation for acupuncture's analgesic effect is that the needles balance and align a patient's life force. But Western physicians, and their Western patients, tend to want Western explanations.

Some suggest that acupuncture's pricks draw the brain's focus from the original source of discomfort. "It's the idea that if your thumb hurts, hit your toe with a hammer," says Mark Lee, chairman of education at Mayo Clinic's Complementary and Integrative Medicine Program. "You won't notice your thumb throbbing because your toe hurts more." The problem with that explanation, Lee says, is that it implies that any needle stuck anywhere should do the trick, and that's not the case.

Others believe that the needles stimulate the body's natural painkillers—called endorphins—and increase blood flow to damaged tissues. These effects are most often associated with electro-acupuncture, in which a light charge is delivered through the needles, causing levels of endorphins and other stress-busting neurochemicals to rise. This explanation doesn't quite stand up to scrutiny either. Lee points out that "even after we remove the needles, the effect remains for some time." Indeed, a 2011 study in rats found that levels of neuropeptide Y—a protein that rises

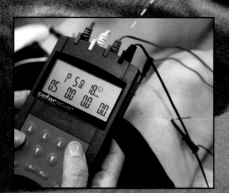

ELECTRO-ACUPUNCTURE: This update of the ancient needlework elevates levels of pain-reducing endorphins and other stress-busting neurochemicals.

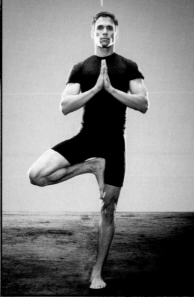

YOGA: Focusing on alignment and strength, this version of the popular workout has been shown to lessen the need for analgesic medication.

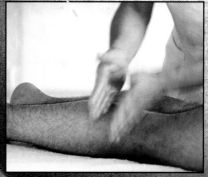

MASSAGE: From fibromyalgia sufferers to patients with post-op discomfort, almost anyone who hurts can benefit from one of the many forms of this hands-on therapy.

in response to stress—remained low for four days after acupuncture.

Still, various neuroimaging techniques show that acupuncture does reduce activity in areas of the brain that process pain. So something is going on; we just haven't yet figured out what or why.

While an understanding of how acupuncture works remains a bit of a mystery, massage is much more a case of what-you-feel-is-what-you-get: Muscles that have been kneaded and stretched hurt less. A 2012 study found that only 10 minutes of massage after vigorous exercise reduced amounts of inflammatory chemicals called cytokines that are produced in the cells of leg muscles. (Inflamed tissues tend to be hypersensitive to painful stimuli; inflammation is the cause not only of injury-related muscle pain, but also of most of the joint pain in arthritis.) Massage also increased production of mitochondria—the organelles that power cells—allowing damaged muscle tissue to spring back to pain-free health quicker.

But massage is no one-rub-fixes-all remedy. Deep-tissue massage, for instance, addresses muscle damage caused by injury. The less forceful Swedish massage primarily relaxes and re-energizes muscles. And trigger-point massage is often ideal for fibromyalgia, a bodywide pain that is more or less defined by the presence of so-called trigger points: unusually sensitive, tight portions of muscle and soft tissue. Massaging these trigger points can increase the range of motion of muscles and joints, and that, in turn, increases the flow of inflammation-dampening (and thus painkilling) white blood cells to affected areas.

Massage can combat more than muscle soreness. A 2007 Mayo study found that pain levels were reduced significantly in patients given massage therapy during recovery from heart surgery; now massage is offered to all of Mayo's cardiac surgery patients. And it can work at the emotional level too. The National Center for Complementary and Alternative Medicine says massage can stimulate the release of endorphins and serotonin to lift mood and reduce the stress and depression that often accompany chronic pain.

"I think most Americans have lost touch with their bodies," says Brent Bauer, director of Mayo Clinic's Integrative Medicine Program. "We aren't aware of how much stress we carry or how that causes, for example, our shoulder muscles to tighten. A good massage sets the stage for reconnecting the mind and body."

One way to accomplish this mind-body connection is yoga—in many ways the premier therapy for pain control. Yoga confers its benefits not just by stretching muscles, but by reducing stress through breath control and the meditative state it can muster. Two different 2011 studies showed yoga to be better than conventional treatments at reducing the impact of pain on patients' functioning. In addition, a 2009 study found that patients needed less pain medication and experienced less depression while performing Iyengar yoga—which focuses on body alignment and strength rather than flexibility and relaxation—most likely because of a neurochemical boost.

Yoga also counters the nonstop ache of fibromyalgia. One recent study found that it significantly decreased pain and increased cortisol levels in women with the condition. (While high cortisol levels are signs of stress in most people, those with fibromyalgia have levels so far below average that it may actually cause their pain and fatigue.) Bauer has also seen benefits in people with carpal tunnel syndrome and those with arthritis of the large joints, like hips and knees.

Yoga is just one of the mind-over-body ways to cripple pain. Guided imagery, the practice of controlled mental visualization, is often used to reduce stress and anxiety, but it also fights pain by refocusing attention. It's the classic exercise: "You're on a white, sandy beach. Waves are crashing onto the shore; the water stretches to the horizon. You're the only person for miles ..." Two recent papers looked at a total of 24 randomized clinical trials—nine of which considered the efficacy of guided imagery on musculoskeletal pain, the other 15 of which looked at non-musculoskeletal pain. Although many of the trials were too small or imperfectly designed to lead researchers to definite conclusions, they called their findings "encouraging." A 2009 study published

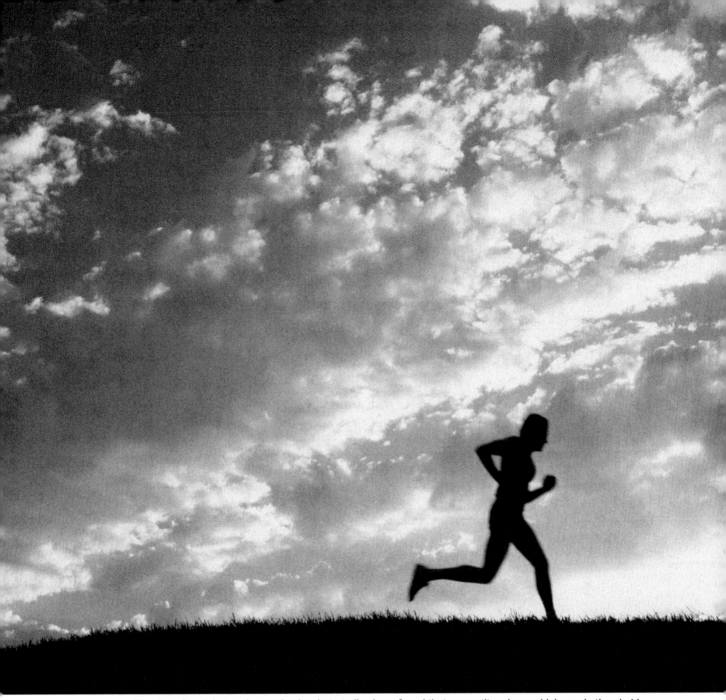

Exercise often brings aches and pains, but studies have found that competitors have a higher pain threshold in comparison to other active adults because they tend to persevere and build up a higher tolerance.

in the journal *Pediatrics* found that children with abdominal pain who listened to audio recordings to guide their visualizations were more than twice as likely to have lower pain levels than kids who used standard treatments—and those benefits persisted for six months.

Because they are easy to use, mind-body therapies work especially well for the elderly. A 2007 review of different interventions found most to be effective in easing their pain. One of those therapies, progressive muscle relaxation, in which you tense and release specific muscle groups in sequence, was particularly effective for osteo-arthritis pain.

Unlike most pain-fighting pharmaceuticals, integrative therapies in general—and mind-body therapies specifically—are virtually free of side effects, as long as they're supervised by licensed, trained practitioners. Better yet, many (guided imagery, meditation) are "pretty accessible to anyone, regardless of socioeconomic status, mobility, and other factors," says Bauer. So what are you waiting for? Pain relief may be just a deep breath or daydream away.

Training Your Mind to Reduce Stress

Our hurried, harried lives can make us sick. By changing the way we think, we can take our brains in a different direction. And where the brain goes, the body tends to follow. **By Alice Park**

WHAT'S THE FIRST THING YOU THINK ABOUT WHEN YOU WAKE UP each morning? Chances are, before you open your eyes you're already focused on the dozens of responsibilities that await you. Maybe your to-do list starts simply, with getting yourself ready for work or packing the kids off to school. But somewhere in those first split seconds you also begin to dread the commute or fret about whether the cable guy is actually going to show up this time. Then there's that nagging pain in your tooth that says you shouldn't put off a visit to the dentist any longer. And don't forget you need to call your mother to see how Dad is doing after hip surgery. You're not even out of bed and you're already mentally exhausted.

As the clutter of thoughts tumbles into consciousness, your physical plant gears up accordingly. Nerve circuits in your brain trip an alarm, letting the rest of your body know that harrying times are ahead. Hormones tip your heart to pump faster. The

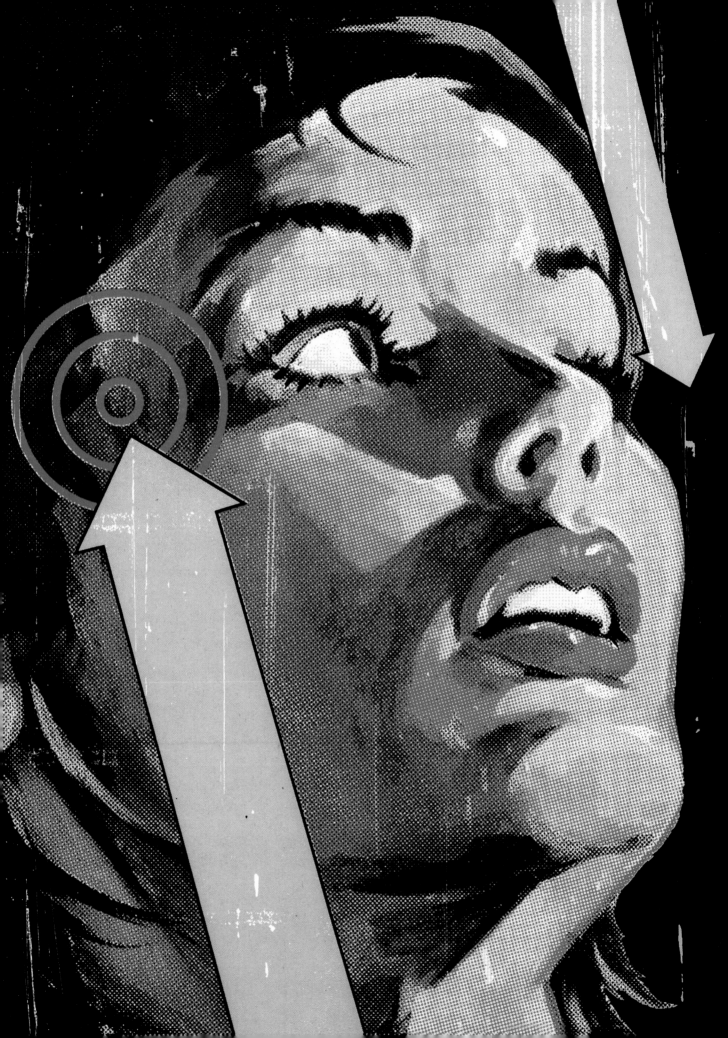

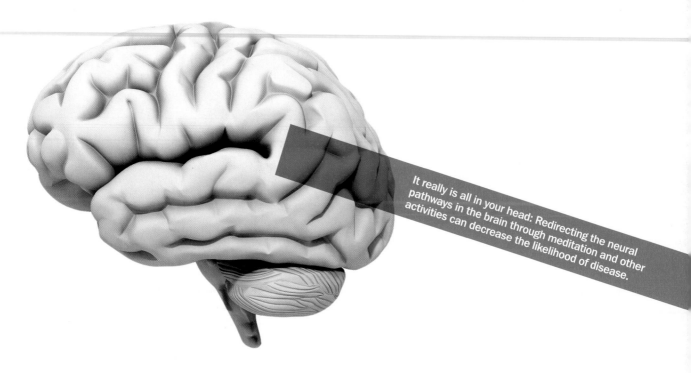

It really is all in your head: Redirecting the neural pathways in the brain through meditation and other activities can decrease the likelihood of disease.

immune system slows its patrol for invading pathogens so that it can cede its share of the body's energy store to other precincts that need to be primed for the impending onslaught. Muscles pull in more oxygen, readying for action. Senses go on high alert.

Somebody might as well have scribbled "Stress was here" across your forehead. And this on a relatively manageable day. Imagine the toll that stress can take over time. Unchecked, those metabolic changes can cause serious ailments, from high blood pressure to obesity to heart disease. Long-term stress also runs down cells, tissues, and organs, making them degenerate before their time. Clearly, when it comes to your fitness, the brain is as important as diet and exercise, because where it goes, the body tends to follow. They say the mind can triumph over matter. Harness it well, and it can beat back sickness too.

As higher-order beings, we worry. We also plan and organize and ruminate: On average, at any given time we are balancing 150 uncompleted tasks and 15 unaccomplished goals. Hence the worrying. These days new technologies allow us to peer behind the knitted brows and twitching eyes to see what that worrying actually looks like. In a 2001 study, researchers at Washington University in St. Louis used functional magnetic resonance imaging (fMRI), which captures real-time changes in oxygen flow in the brain during mental tasks, to map a baseline state of cranial activity. They found that the amount of oxygen expended during many routine chores—reading, for example—is actually comparable to the amount dispersed during eyes-closed rest. But the portrait the MRI painted of a brain working to tie up a bunch of loose ends—a brain mired in stress—looked very different. A brain in the process of serially ticking off the upcoming day's to-do list activates a particular circuit of neurons that loops in the hypothalamus, pituitary, and adrenal glands and triggers the release of the hormones cortisol and adrenaline, both of which set the body on edge. Like a pebble dropped in a pond, this turned-on circuit then sends tension throughout the body, pushing a variety of metabolic systems off balance. It's why your heart races and your hands get damp, why a knot grows in your stomach and your chest tightens.

We all know too well how easy it is to turn this stress system on. Turning it off … well, that's something else entirely. Turns out, toggling your brain between a pattern of agitation and one of calm isn't like flipping a switch at all. How could it be? What we're talking about, after all, is nothing less than manipulating molecular pathways that link the brain's infinitely complex network of 100 billion nerve cells with virtually every other

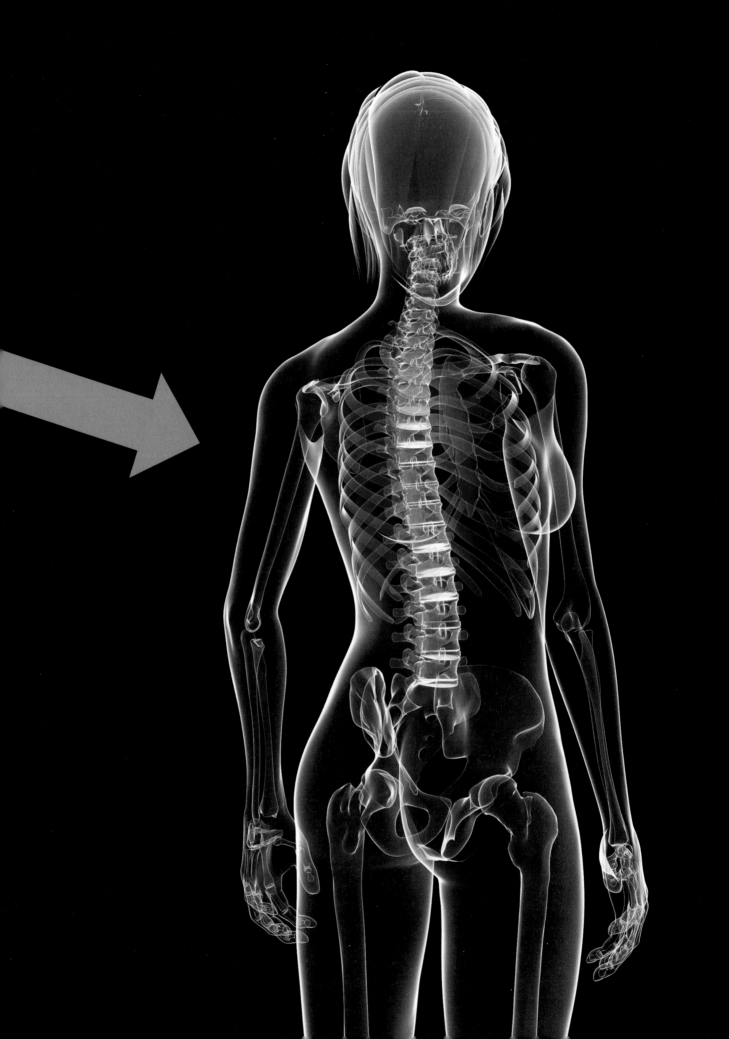

tissue and organ in the body. There is no remote control for that.

There are, however, other ways to change your channel. As head of the Stress Management and Resiliency Training (SMART) Program at Mayo Clinic, Amit Sood gives participants concrete ways to accomplish just that. But before he puts his mind-body medicine into practice, he showers them with science. "If you want to learn about stress management and resilience, you need to know about the brain," Sood says. He begins by describing two different modes of the brain. One is activated when a person focuses on external events or tasks, like finishing a puzzle, appreciating a painting, or getting lost in a song. The other is the product of internalized thoughts: planning, thinking, and worrying. Those internalized thoughts are where trouble lies.

Everything that competes for our attention, he explains, falls into one of three categories: threat, pleasure, or novelty. And unfortunately we have evolved to prioritize threat. That's how early man protected himself from mortal dangers like predators, flood, and fire. Today most of the threats we encounter are of our own making, such as anxiety about upcoming engagements, guilt over things we have done or said, and fears of the future. At first glance, those "threats" don't seem to pack the menace of a hungry sabertooth cat. But they engulf our attention like black holes all the same. And once we are sucked in, it's extremely difficult to free ourselves from the gravitational pull.

Making escape even more sticky is the fact that a stressful state often becomes the brain's default setting, one it slips into almost automatically. Blame human biology. Like a gymtrained muscle, the plasticity

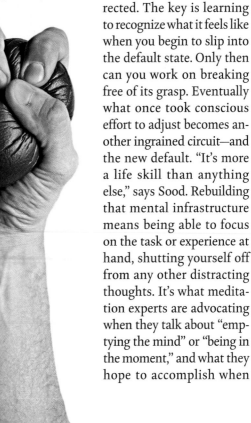

of the brain allows its frequently used nerves and networks to grow stronger too. So over time, familiar pathways become well worn, like a rutted country road, and your thoughts end up stuck following routes that take them somewhere other than where you want them to go. Soon, obsessing over perceived threats is your norm; you go to bed with your head spinning with them and wake up still churning. "This is nobody's fault; it's ingrained in the way these networks are set up," Sood says.

The stress response was always meant to be an emergency measure only, a quick and focused response to impending and immediate disaster. But modern-day threats—job security, your faltering 401(k), your daughter's new boyfriend—tend to linger. And neither our brains nor our bodies were designed to manage that kind of sustained strain. So they protest. And that rebellion takes the form of heart disease, hypertension, stroke, and depression.

Fortunately—and here is the point of Sood's training—just as those well-worn negative neural pathways can be created, they can also be redirected. The key is learning to recognize what it feels like when you begin to slip into the default state. Only then can you work on breaking free of its grasp. Eventually what once took conscious effort to adjust becomes another ingrained circuit—and the new default. "It's more a life skill than anything else," says Sood. Rebuilding that mental infrastructure means being able to focus on the task or experience at hand, shutting yourself off from any other distracting thoughts. It's what meditation experts are advocating when they talk about "emptying the mind" or "being in the moment," and what they hope to accomplish when

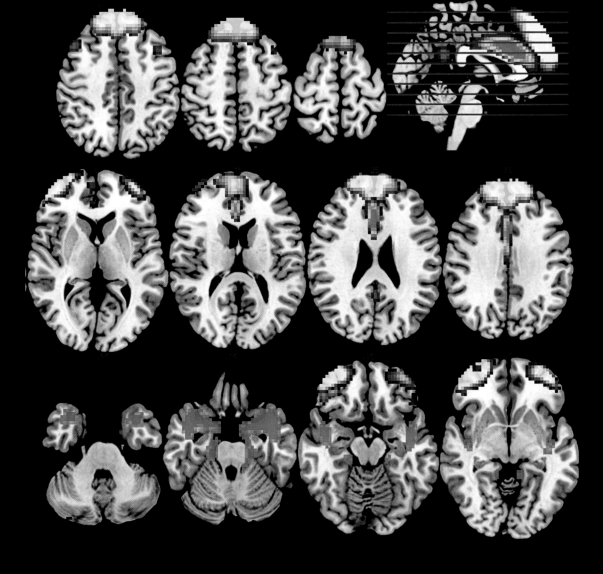

This is what worry looks like: By using color to demonstrate the flow of oxygen, fMRIs (brain scans) capture changes in different brains as their owners rest, and then as they start to consider the problems of the day. Once that process begins, neurons are activated that spread tension throughout the rest of the body. This can eventually lead to high blood pressure, stroke, heart disease, and depression.

they ask clients to concentrate on their breathing. Of course, the more ingrained the stress pathway, the more difficult this seemingly uncomplicated task can be.

Sood says you just have to train your brain one thought at a time. Be more attentive to external rather than internal experiences. Start with those very first thoughts of the morning. Don't be ensnared by responsibilities; welcome the day instead by thinking about five loved ones. Picturing their faces one at a time, remind yourself why you are grateful and happy to have them in your life.

Then, throughout the day, take 10-minute breaks to draw yourself away from your pressure-filled routines. When you're with friends or family members, treat them as if you are meeting after a long time apart; pay attention to what they say and how they are feeling. Sometimes a change of scenery helps, so take a walk. Make sure it's not a march to the finish, though, consumed all the while by the chaos in your head. The purpose of getting away is to get away.

Oh, and if on one of your strolls, you happen to stop by a rosebush, you know what to do.

After Surgery: Let the Healing Begin

A new hospital program offers treatments that help relieve the physical, mental, and emotional problems that often accompany surgical procedures. **By Jeffrey Kluger**

AN OPERATING ROOM IS A MONUMENT TO THE IDEA OF NOT MESSING around. Nobody schedules surgery by accident or just for fun. When you deliver yourself into the hands of semi-strangers and give them license—indeed, pay them money—to knock you out, open you up, and manipulate your very innards, you want to know there is hard science on your side.

That's one reason complementary and alternative medicine (CAM) has had such a rough time gaining purchase in most pre- and post-surgical wards. Even as more than 40% of Americans report receiving some kind of CAM treatment in any given year, the surgical arena has long been off-limits. A drum circle and a hug won't cut it once you've moved into the world of scalpels, sutures, and drills; at that point you want drugs, scans, computers, blood tests—the multimillion-dollar empirical stuff that's been proved to work.

The problem is, hard science and clinical reason can take you only so far, because human beings are decidedly messy creatures. Surgery isn't just about repairing or re-

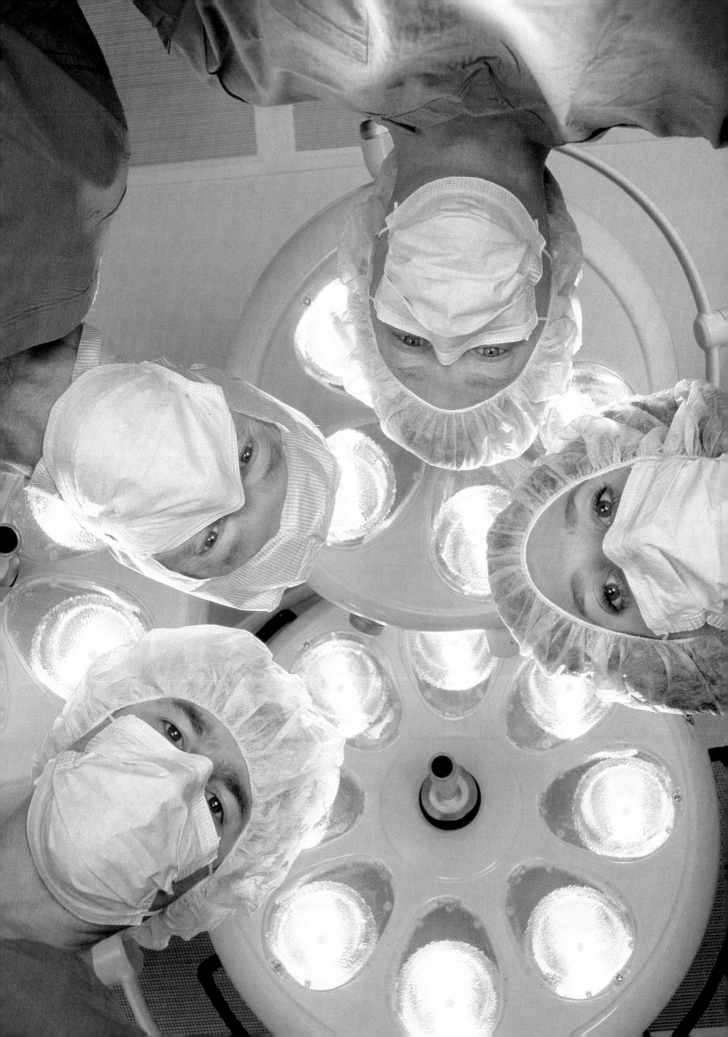

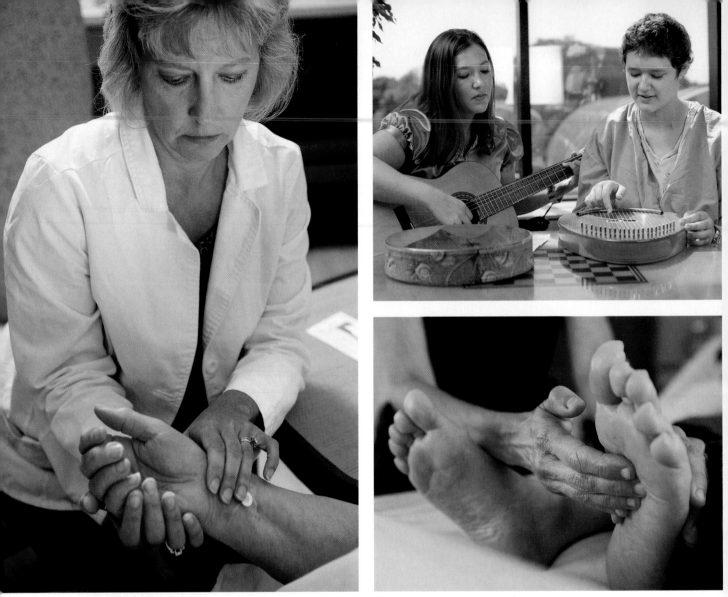

From left: Acupressure may help relieve nausea; a music therapist joins a young woman as she expresses her medical journey through tunes; and reflexology is a good pre- or post-surgical relaxation effect.

moving sick tissue—it's about fear, pain, depression, and stress, not to mention the deep existential terror that comes from walking into a hospital and knowing there's a risk that you may not walk out again. That's not the kind of thing that can be diagnosed with a CT scan or treated with a microsurgical robot. But it is exactly the kind of thing that can have a significant impact on healing.

In 2006 the American Academy of Orthopaedic Surgeons published a meta-analysis of 14 years' worth of studies showing that what doctors call "psychosocial factors" and everyone else calls "feeling lousy and depressed" can have a powerful effect on how quickly surgical patients recover and how successful their surgery turns out to be. A 2009 study from Melbourne, Australia, found the same results in coronary bypass

surgery, as did a 2001 U.K. analysis that looked at 20 years of recovery records for all surgical procedures.

Studies like those have pushed more leading medical institutions to look for new ways to improve the patient experience—never mind if those ways aren't quite what we've grown to expect. Almost a decade ago, Mayo Clinic made one of the first big pushes into incorporating CAM into its pre- and post-op wards, targeting cardiac patients specifically. Few procedures are as grueling as heart surgery. For all the advances made in minimally invasive cardiac care—with stents, angioplasty balloons, and other instruments threaded through an artery in the groin up to the heart—some procedures are still done the old-fashioned way. There's just no other means to replace a valve or perform a bypass, for

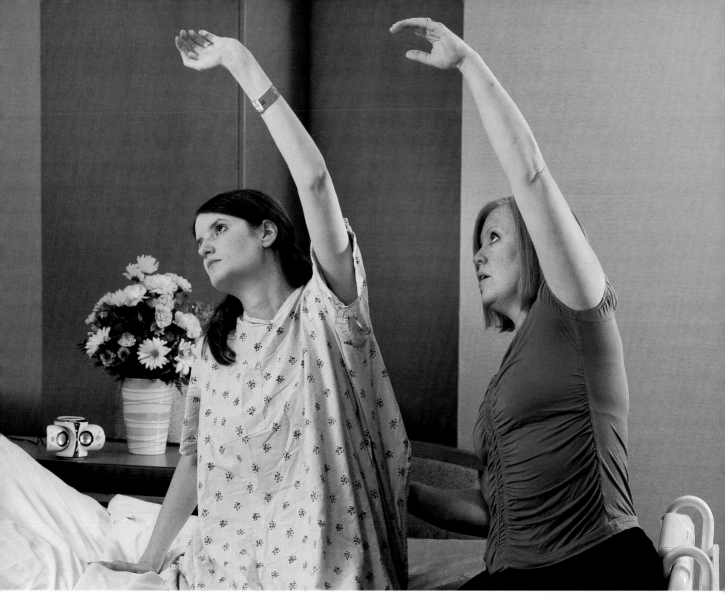

At Mayo, patients increasingly ask for post-surgical yoga, which the clinic offers at bedside.

example, than by cutting the sternum, splitting the chest, and subjecting the patient to hours of deep anesthesia while the heart is manipulated by hand, scalpel, and suture. And yet the inevitable post-surgical suffering goes beyond the trauma the chest has sustained.

"Patients experience pain for a lot of reasons," says Susanne Cutshall, a nursing instructor and Mayo Clinic integrative health specialist. "There's pain from the long hours spent on the table, there's pain from the unfamiliar hospital bed. There's pain, too, simply from holding so much tension and from what's known as guarding behavior—positioning yourself differently after surgery to protect tubes and lines."

All that awfulness makes feeling better—not to mention actually getting better—difficult. Mayo researchers thus decided to determine

whether a bit of massage might help the healing process along. Recruiting 58 patients before they underwent surgery, the researchers assigned 30 to receive standard post-surgical care—including pain medications—plus two 20-minute sessions of massage on the second and fifth days after surgery. The remaining 28 received the same care, except they spent those 20 minutes quietly relaxing with no massage.

Both before and after the sessions, the patients evaluated their level of pain, anxiety, and tension on what's known as a visual analog scale—a fancy way of saying they used a diagram to rate how good or bad they felt, from 1 to 10. All the subjects in the Mayo study started out in more or less the same range—anywhere from 4.5 to 8 in all three categories. But after just 20 minutes of hands-on attention, the massage group

Massages help to lessen pain and improve sleep for patients who have undergone surgery.

fell to a 1.0 for anxiety, 1.8 for pain, and 2.0 for tension. The control group weighed in at 4.5, 4.2, and 4.5, respectively.

More important than the numbers, though, was how the patients talked about the experience. "This was the best thing since the surgery," said one. "I finally had a good night's sleep," said another. These were just the reactions the investigators were looking for. "There were some positive data points from the studies," says Cutshall. "But the biggest thing was what the patients said. That sealed it."

There have been similar results for audio-therapy—simply listening to music or recorded nature sounds to reduce post-surgical pain and anxiety. In a 2011 study, Mayo researchers recruited 100 patients recovering from heart surgery and divided them roughly in half, with one group listening to soothing recordings for 20 minutes per day on days two through four post-surgery and the other simply relaxing. As with the massage study, the results were definitive: While both groups came out of the OR with equivalent levels of pain—roughly 3 on a 1-to-10 scale—by day four, the music group was down to less than 1.5. The non-music group, meanwhile, actually rose slightly, to about 3.25. Anxiety scores were similar, if a bit less dramatic, with the music listeners averaging just 0.8, and the others clocking in at about 1.6. Findings like these have an impact on more than just a patient's well-being during a hospital stay. Multiple studies have shown that people whose pain is dealt with quickly and effectively tend to recover faster than those who have a less comfortable time in the immediate post-op days.

Agonizing as pain can be, many patients coming out of surgery suffer even more from nausea. It's a common side effect of general anesthesia that can be exacerbated by drugs or even the stress of being hospitalized. In 2009, Mayo doctors wanted to learn if acupuncture administered 30 minutes to three hours before surgery could prevent or at least reduce nausea. Once again, they recruited a group and administered acupuncture to half of the patients. Once again, the unconventional methods worked: The subjects

who received acupuncture reported feeling nauseous significantly less frequently than the other group, and their suffering was significantly less acute when they did feel ill. "A single pre-operative acupuncture treatment reduced incidence and severity ... and caused no adverse effects," the study's authors wrote.

It's not just patients who can benefit from CAM techniques. Members of the nursing staff—the ground forces of the surgical wing—have enjoyed a benefit from alternative methods. In one study Cutshall conducted in 2011, nurses who used a biofeedback computer program to practice relaxation techniques four times a week for four weeks experienced less stress and exhibited fewer signs of burnout than a control group. That's no small advantage in a modern medical environment in which a third to half of all nurses in intensive- or critical-care units suffer from fatigue, anxiety, or depression, or exhibit other signs of severe burnout.

All along the line, patients have gotten similar benefits from other, equally non-mainstream treatments. Aromatherapy—with spearmint, peppermint, ginger, or lavender oils—has been shown to ease post-op nausea. Reiki—a sort of laying-on of hands—has reduced stress and sped healing. Patients in the Mayo network are also offered meditation, yoga, tai chi, and even animal therapy, in which companion dogs visit patients before and after surgery. More to the point, people are increasingly requesting those services. In 2011, Mayo reached 20,000 patients and family members with various complementary therapies.

That number is likely to grow—and not just at Mayo. The uniquely violative, uniquely mortal nature of surgery makes it a feared and serious enterprise. But such gravity can open minds and clarify thinking too. Wisdom dictates not accepting just any old nostrum. Wisdom also dictates embracing ideas you might not ordinarily consider. When your health, welfare, and life are on the line, you're not likely to be picky about where legitimate help comes from. Relief and recovery are what count—and, more and more, CAM is delivering both.

Society of the Healing Heart

To get the word out about a long-silent epidemic, women with heart disease tell their stories like health-care evangelists. By Alice Park

ONE WEEK. THAT'S HOW LONG IT TOOK RHONDA MONROE TO GET CONfirmation of what she already knew. While laying her 5-day-old daughter in her crib, Monroe felt a sudden tightness in her chest ("It was like an elephant was sitting there") and broke out in a sweat. She sensed what was happening, and when she called 911, the EMTs agreed: It was a heart attack. At the hospital, the doctors took one look at her—she was 36, not overweight, and otherwise healthy—and sent her home. She went, but when the pain and tingling in her arms didn't go away, she returned to the ER. They sent her away again, this time with some pain medicine. Monroe continued to wake up each morning with the same heavy feeling. She visited her primary physician, an urgent-care center, then the hospital again. After five days, she finally found a cardiologist who got it right.

If only staying healthy were as simple as eating a nutritious diet, getting enough exercise, and sleeping well. Fighting off disease, though, means also arming yourself

with the knowledge to recognize a problem when it rears up—and how to take preventive action before it does. Neglecting to take the time to get that education can be a potentially fatal mistake. But even if, like Monroe, you are not uninformed, getting the help you need can be difficult.

To be fair, women's heart disease is a tricky business. Monroe's story shows that even getting an accurate diagnosis can be a challenge, complicated by certain unyielding realities that affect not only patients but doctors as well. Some are shockingly basic. "Many physicians don't even know that more women than men die of heart disease," notes Sharonne Hayes, a cardiologist at Mayo Clinic.

The sad truth is, otherwise diligent doctors often miss heart attacks in women simply because they aren't looking for them. It doesn't help that women's heart attacks often manifest differently from men's, lacking the pair of classic symptoms: chest pain and shortness of breath. Instead, the pain is typically more diffuse, radiating through the back or shoulders rather than bearing down on the chest. Further, women tend to develop heart trouble a decade later than men do, in their sixties and seventies, at which time doctors have already begun to focus on other explanations for symptoms. The upshot is that stricken women aren't treated quickly enough, making heart disease the leading cause of death among U.S. females. Worse, 42% die within a year of suffering a heart attack, compared with 24% of men, in large part because the disease in women, having gone untreated, is typically more advanced.

In 2002, Hayes began to think about how to combat this serious gender inequality. Her instincts told her that a grassroots campaign was the way to go. If physicians weren't adopting—or even acknowledging—the latest wisdom about women's heart disease, maybe cutting out the middleman and bringing the message straight to the people at risk would produce better results. "I felt we needed to build awareness with our boots on the ground," Hayes says. So she and three of her patients hatched an idea.

As one of WomenHeart's earliest participants and educators, Monroe tells her death-defying story everywhere women will listen—in this case, at a beauty salon in West Virginia.

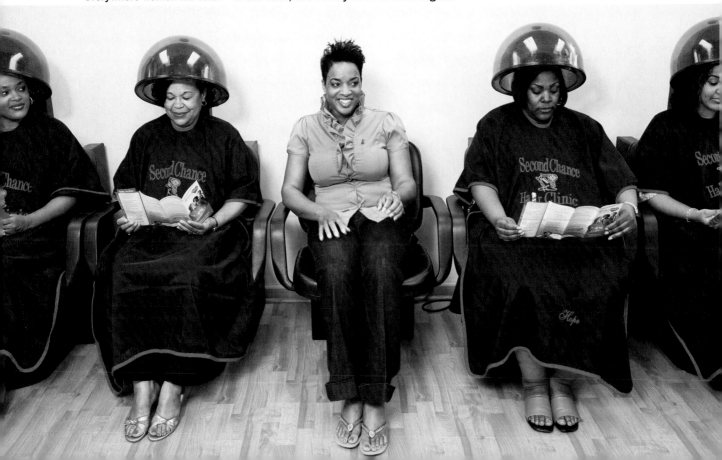

They developed WomenHeart, a program specifically geared to women with heart disease, and built on the theory that support groups and education are powerful allies in the promotion of health. There is a good precedent in breast cancer management. The extensive networks of breast cancer survivors, through which they share experiences and advice with newly diagnosed peers, have not only improved screening rates but also put a dent in the incidence of the disease.

At the first WomenHeart sessions, it was immediately evident that the gap Hayes was looking to bridge was vast. Not one attendee had ever met another woman with heart disease. At the same time, most had a harrowing tale to share of being misdiagnosed or dismissed altogether by doctors who didn't even consider the possibility of heart disease.

Today participants come from all over the U.S., recruited by word of mouth from patients treated at Mayo Clinic. Each year, several dozen women gather at the clinic in Rochester, Minn., leaving behind full-time jobs and families for a few days of healthful indoctrination. All are cardiac survivors—women who have had heart attacks, heart surgeries, heart failures, or a combination. All are motivated to help others avoid the same fate. Monroe, it turns out, was one of WomenHeart's earliest participants. As is the tradition, she shared her story with the group.

As soon as the cardiologist diagnosed her heart attack, he scheduled a quadruple bypass. But the damage done during the week Monroe went undiagnosed caused many complications. She developed pericarditis, an inflammation of the sac that encases the heart, and congestive heart failure. Today she has an implanted defibrillator to keep her heart pumping when it gets sluggish. Eight months after her bypass, the blood vessels that had been grafted onto her heart to keep blood flowing shut down, requiring another operation. "I've been told over and over that I wouldn't have the problems I have now if they'd listened to me then," she says. "So I tell women whenever I can that if they are feeling any pain in their chest, they need to take it seriously and be persistent."

Taking a cue from breast cancer awareness groups, WomenHeart participants in Plano, Texas, have adopted a symbol, red knit HeartScarves, to raise awareness about cardiovascular disease.

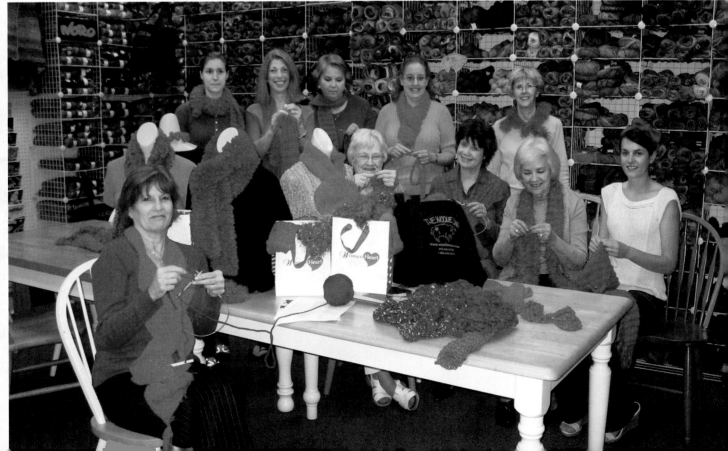

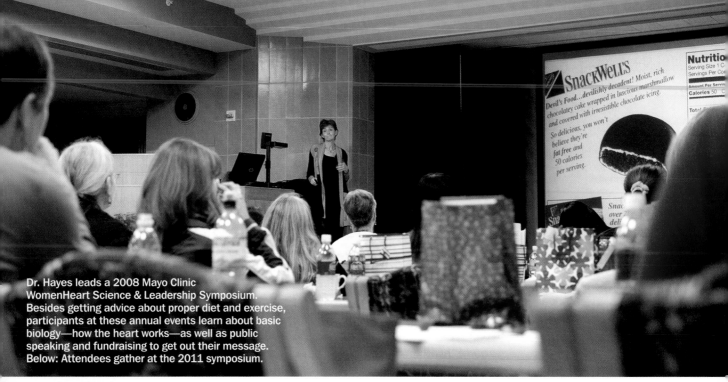

Dr. Hayes leads a 2008 Mayo Clinic
WomenHeart Science & Leadership Symposium.
Besides getting advice about proper diet and exercise,
participants at these annual events learn about basic
biology—how the heart works—as well as public
speaking and fundraising to get out their message.
Below: Attendees gather at the 2011 symposium.

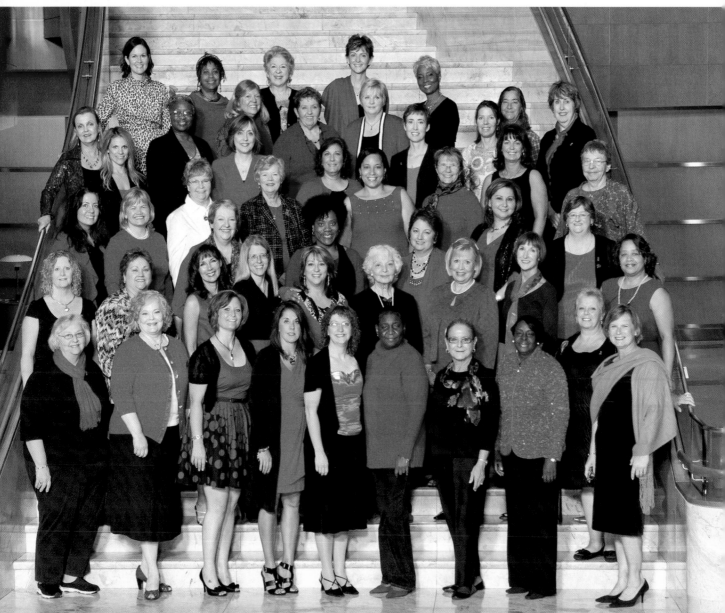

The story told by Suzie Arnegger is shockingly similar to Monroe's. Arnegger, a claims adjuster in San Diego, spent six months shuttling back and forth among seven doctors and two emergency rooms seeking help for a pain that spread across her eyes and into her jaw, not to mention recurring nausea. Her symptoms led physicians to suspect everything from migraines to menopause. Everything but the correct diagnosis: heart disease. On a morning when her pain was particularly bad, Arnegger drove to a local urgent-care clinic. When she got there, it had not yet opened, so she turned her car around and headed home. Stopped at a red light, she noticed a hospital and decided to give it a try, but an emergency-room doctor simply ordered a round of gastrointestinal tests and left her alone. And that's when it hit. "My arms and legs went from tingling to numb, and fast—boom, boom, boom," Arnegger says. "It was so sudden and severe that the doctor said if I'd been at home, I wouldn't have made it." She calls it her drive-by heart attack.

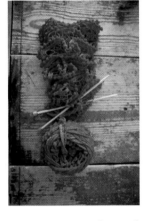

Hayes and her team guide women to the universal lessons that can be gleaned from such experiences, lessons they can take home to their neighborhoods and towns. WomenHeart sessions also include basic biology—how the heart works, what goes wrong during an attack—and training in public speaking, fundraising, and how to approach hospitals and community centers for resources and potential participants.

Arnegger is one of hundreds of WomenHeart champions, as graduates of the program are called, working to spread the word. In 2006, in her new hometown of Plano, Texas, she and a fellow training mate launched HeartScarves, a program in which women knit red scarves for patients who are undergoing heart procedures or recovering from heart disease. The pair have hundreds of knitters clicking needles to raise awareness.

Each champion advocates in her own way. Some women appear on TV. Others run fundraisers to support research and educational programs. Still others build support groups and special rehabilitation programs specifically for women with heart disease. In Charles Town, W.Va., where Monroe now lives, she holds forth at places like a friend's beauty salon. After telling her story and conducting a Q&A session there, she was asked back for an encore.

That's exactly the kind of response Hayes envisioned when she began WomenHeart. Health, she says, isn't achieved just by treating disease when it happens but by being smarter about recognizing and combatting its precursors. And proselytizing cardiac survivors can accomplish far more than doctors can during an office visit. "We're focused on turning awareness into action," Hayes says.

The action can be as simple as calling 911, which women are less likely to do than men, even when they are in pain. And that's a problem that advocates can address more effectively than any physician, by telling their stories and providing real-life examples of how a single call can save their lives. The support groups also seek to free women from the guilt that comes with their heart disease, the belief that their failing tickers are a result of poor lifestyle choices. "A lot of women blame themselves for their condition," says Hayes, "especially women in competitive jobs."

It doesn't hurt when celebrities lend their support as well. When comedian Rosie O'Donnell suffered a heart attack in August 2012, she immediately blogged this advice to women: "Know the symptoms ladies," she wrote. "Listen to the voice inside, the one we all so easily ignore. CALL 911."

In the best-case scenario, says Hayes, the program she started becomes obsolete as patients and doctors alike know enough to keep women safe. Until then, she will continue to tend to the heartbeat of her program, pushing to make it stronger and stronger.

A version of this story originally appeared in TIME *magazine.*

Nothing To Sneeze At

It's true: Global warming is making seasonal allergies worse than ever. Turns out, some of the best weapons against this itchy future may be ancient ones. By Bryan Walsh

T HE SPRING OF 2012 WAS A GREAT ONE FOR FANS OF PRETERNATURALLY warm weather and prematurely budding flowers, significantly less so for any of the roughly 40% of Americans who suffer from seasonal allergies. An unusually warm and dry winter across much of the U.S., followed by the hottest March on record, ushered in an especially early spring, and this particular version came loaded with unusually high levels of tree pollen. The result, according to the National Allergy Bureau, which tracks these microscopic irritants, was an allergy season shifted forward a month. And that meant millions of Americans found themselves sneezing and sniffling, blowing their noses, and dabbing at watery eyes well ahead of schedule. As Alvin Sanico of Johns Hopkins Hospital says, "People were caught by surprise."

Nature's global-warming-induced practical joke is just the latest reminder of how tough allergies can be to control. Americans already spend more than $30 billion each

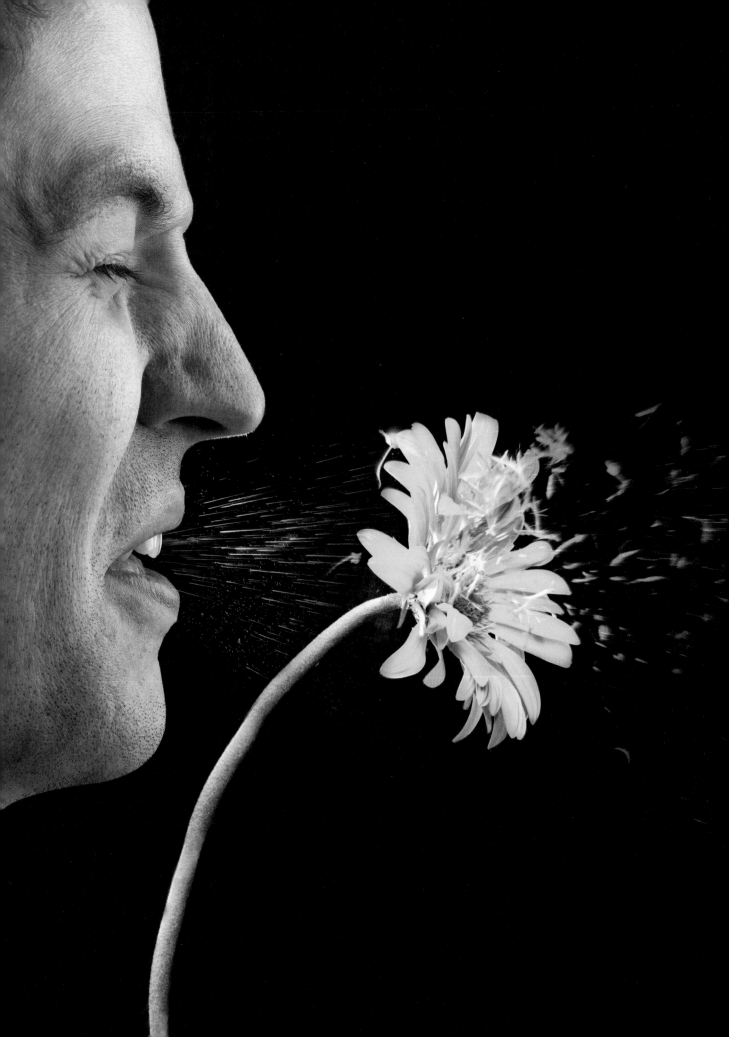

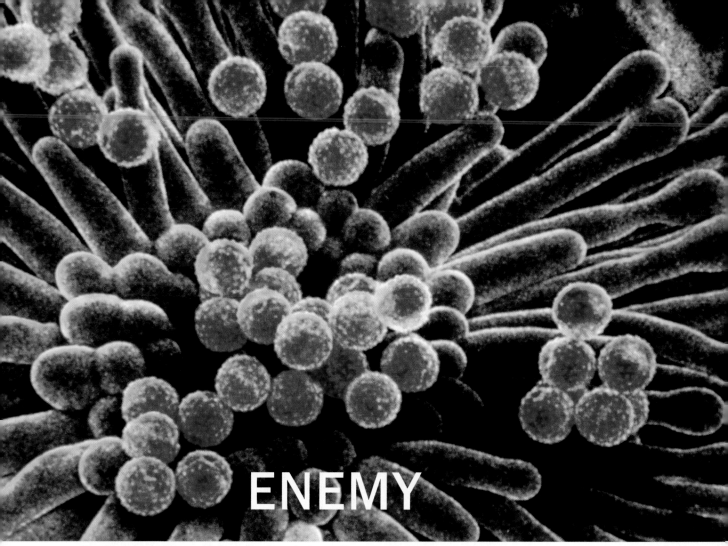

ENEMY

The 41 species of ragweed, flowering plants in the sunflower family, are notorious for the severe allergies caused by their pollen.

year on allergy and asthma care. On the day the antihistamine Allegra became available over the counter in 2012, manufacturers shipped more than 8 million pills. And now we can't even predict when hay fever and its vexing relatives will come knocking? Something that is so common, so annoying, and so unpredictable is bound to have desperate victims seeking relief wherever they can find it. In fact, allergy sufferers have been quick to turn to alternative-medicine options in significant numbers—upwards of one in four of them, according to a 2011 study. But the question, as always, is: Are any of those treatments more than false hope in a bottle?

The short answer is yes, particularly if that answer includes "butterbur." Butterbur is an herb whose roots were made into a remedy for headaches and inflammation by Native Americans. Today you can buy tablets of it over the counter. In a 2002 study published in the *British Medi-*

cal Journal, Swiss researchers showed that one tablet taken four times daily can be as effective as the popular antihistamine cetirizine (brand name: Zyrtec) in controlling symptoms of hay fever—and without the drowsiness that's often associated with this kind of traditional allergy medicine. Another study found that butterbur worked as well as the antihistamine fexofenadine (Allegra) at relieving sneezing, congestion, and itchy eyes.

Like conventional antihistamines, butterbur seems to block the effects of histamine and leukotrienes, those inflammatory chemicals that are activated by allergens and trigger the runny noses and watery eyes that every hay fever sufferer dreads. Another substance called quercetin, a natural antioxidant, works in a similar way. Quercetin appears in some foods, like red apples, but it, too, is available in supplement form (typical dose: 200 to 400 milligrams, three times a day).

FRIEND

Butterbur has been used for more than 1,000 years to treat runny noses caused by allergies; it works by inhibiting the inflammatory compounds histamine and leukotrienes.

Other natural remedies that have been found to offer some relief include stinging nettle—which you can eat like spinach or consume in capsules or tea—and goldenseal, an herb with quite a memorable nickname: "king of the mucous membranes." "King" may be a bit strong, but goldenseal does reduce inflammation and mucus production in the eyes, sinuses, nose, and throat. Avoid it, though, if you have cardiovascular problems—berberine, one of the herb's active ingredients, can disrupt heart rhythms. Pregnant and breastfeeding women need to stay away from it, and infants given goldenseal have developed a rare but serious neurological condition known as kernicterus.

Girding against the seasonal onslaught of allergens isn't just a matter of what you ingest. Hay fever victims and other weed pollen sufferers can benefit from what they don't put in their bodies. Melon, cucumber, banana, chamomile, and supplements that contain echinacea—a popular herbal treatment for colds and other respiratory infections—can often trigger the same allergic reactions that ragweed pollen does. In fact, echinacea is a member of the same botanical family as ragweed. By the way, echinacea doesn't even seem to do what it is supposed to do—prevent or alleviate colds—according to a 2005 study in the *New England Journal of Medicine.*

Herbal medicines and dietary restrictions fall woefully short when your head is a cement block of congestion, however. Many clogged sufferers are inclined to head straight for a decongestant nasal spray or pill, but they can come with side effects like drowsiness, and even worsen symptoms if they're used more than three days in a row. An old-time alternative—the Neti pot—may be a better solution. Resembling a small plastic teapot and usually selling for around $10—the Neti pot makes it easy to snort warm saline water, which irrigates the sinus cavity and shrinks the sinus walls, thus relieving congestion. A 2007 study at the University of Michigan found that adults with chronic nasal and sinus problems who were treated with irrigation had better results over a two-month period than those on a conventional spray. It has reduced the need for steroid sprays in kids with allergies too. Just be sure to boil the water first—there have been reports of infections from the use of unfiltered tap water in Neti pots. "Nasal irrigation—including using Neti pots—was very popular" decades ago, says Brent Bauer, director of Mayo Clinic's Complementary and Integrative Medicine Program. "It turns out to be fairly effective for a lot of mild nasal symptoms, with fewer side effects than many of the medications and sprays."

Common sense says the best allergy treatment—alternative or otherwise—would be to avoid whatever irritant causes the problem. Few doctors would counsel a hay fever sufferer to take a stroll through a cloud of pollen. But you may have heard of an alternative treatment known as homeopathy, which is actually built on the

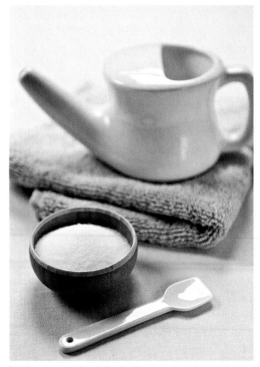

Neti pots, used to irrigate the nasal cavity and reduce irritation, have made a comeback.

theory that "like cures like"—that is, consuming a bit of a substance that causes disease in healthy people can cure that disease in the sick. Conventional practitioners regard homeopathy with a skeptical eye, and you can't blame them. With active ingredients in these remedies diluted by as much as 99%, it does seem a stretch to think they could have much of a medical effect. And few if any placebo-controlled studies have proved otherwise.

A more reasonable alternative is acupuncture. The ancient Chinese medical art is better known as a treatment for pain, as the piercing needles signal the brain to release morphine-like neurotransmitters known as endorphins. But endorphins may also help people with asthma or hay fever breathe easier. In a 2004 study published in the journal *Pediatrics*, school-age allergy sufferers who underwent a regular course of acupuncture had better symptom scores and more symptom-free days—both during treatment and afterward—than those given a placebo acupuncture therapy. (The placebo treatment involved the insertion of needles to much shallower depths than with actual acupuncture.) It's notable that the kids in the study said they preferred oral medications to acupuncture—probably because not everyone is eager to be poked with needles. Also, aside from this one, studies that show a significant benefit to allergy sufferers from acupuncture are rare.

As people with allergies know all too well, "significant benefit" is often too much to ask for. Like the common cold, seasonal allergies can only be managed; they are never really defeated. That was demoralizing enough before recent climatic realities ramped things up. Early springs surprise us now, but they're likely to be routine before long, so seasonal allergies are almost certainly going to worsen. And premature discomfort is just the half of it: A recent study in the *Proceedings of the National Academy of Sciences* showed a strong link between increasing temperatures and a longer ragweed pollen season.

But, then, all the wet, red eyes staring at this page seem to say that this isn't exactly news.

Allergist's Restaurant: A Dining Guide

Diet can make a difference for just about every health condition, so why should allergies be an exception? Here are five foods that have been shown to minimize the agony of seasonal sufferers—while boosting overall health as well.

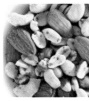 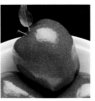   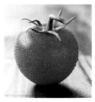

Nuts

A 2007 study found that children from the island of Crete who ate a Mediterranean diet —fresh fruits and vegetables, fish, olive oil, nuts— were less likely to develop allergy and asthma symptoms. Explaining the first four items is easy: Studies show that a diet high in antioxidants (fruits, veggies, olive oil) and omega-3 fatty acids (fish) can ease seasonal allergy suffering. But what do nuts have to do with it? Well, they are rich in magnesium, which helps protect against the wheezing that accompanies asthma, and vitamin E, which boosts immunity and protects against free radicals, those floating molecules that cause inflammation.

Apples

In that same Crete diet study, researchers found that people whose diets included apples as a staple had greater protection against both allergies and asthma. Apples are rich in quercetin, a flavonoid with anti-inflammatory properties. But don't peel them— much of the benefit comes from the skin, which is also packed with antioxidants called polyphenols that help prevent cell damage. Another study found that pregnant women who ate apples reduced the risk of their children developing asthma. Kids whose moms ate the most apples during pregnancy were the least likely to report wheezing or to have asthma at age 5.

Fish

Omega-3 fatty acids in seafood have natural anti-inflammatory effects that boost the immune system—which is helpful, given that allergies occur when your immune system is out of whack. In the study of pregnant apple eaters, researchers also found that expectant moms who ate fish during pregnancy also reduced the risk of their children developing asthma or allergic diseases. The kids whose moms ate fish once a week or more were less likely to have eczema than children of mothers who never ate fish. Not a fan of fish? Try omega-3 and algae supplements or fish oil to boost your defenses.

Grapes

The skin of red grapes is high in antioxidants and resveratrol, another anti-inflammatory compound. Reducing inflammation throughout the body can go a long way toward lowering the impact of allergies. It also helps reduce the risk of heart disease and other cardiovascular problems, which have been connected to inflammation. Stick with red grapes, though. Green, purple, white, blush ... no other color is as rich in either antioxidants or resveratrol.

Tomatoes

Fruity vegetables like tomatoes are high in vitamin C, and studies say that can help build tolerance against asthma and respiratory problems. Vitamin C is an immune system booster and natural antihistamine, but it also suppresses swelling. Plus, tomatoes contain lycopene, another antioxidant compound. A study from the University of Tel Aviv found that men who added 30 milligrams of lycopene to their daily diet improved their ability to fight off asthma attacks by 45%. In another study, Spanish children who consumed more than 40 grams of fruity veggies a day—including eggplant, cucumber, and zucchini—were much less likely to suffer from childhood asthma than those who ate less.

Plants With Benefits

Plants were the original medicines. Long before FDA-approved pharmaceuticals and synthetic vitamins, people relied on leaves, seeds, and flowers as the best lines of defense against illness. Every culture had its favorites, and we can learn something from each. However, many have yet to be subjected to rigorous study, so we still don't know how safe and effective they are, both in general and to each individual with his or her particular needs. Ancient claims are not the same as scientific proof. Before adding any herbal product to your routine, do your research about possible side effects and interactions it might have with prescription drugs. And consult your caregivers before taking the plunge.

Graphic designed by Anne-Michelle Gallero

AYURVEDIC

Ayurveda, "the study of life," is a Hindu system that dates to 300 BCE. Taking into account personality, pulse, and habits, it is the original holistic approach. In India, 80% of the population still practices Ayurveda, but its complexity and controversy (some of its herbs contain toxins) keep it outside the Western mainstream.

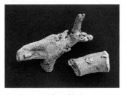

Ashwagandha
"That which has the smell of a horse" is said to offer the vitality and sexual energy of a stallion.

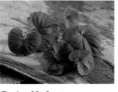

Gotu Kola
Used to revitalize nerves and brain cells, and thus to supposedly increase intelligence, memory, and longevity.

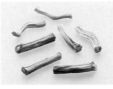

Shatavari Also known as asparagus root (not to be confused with the vegetable we eat), it is seen as a major rejuvenative tonic for women. Used for fertility and menopause problems.

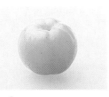

Amla
One of these walnut-size fruits has the vitamin C of 10 oranges.

CHINESE

Another ancient holistic system that continues to evolve, though herbal remedies and acupuncture remain its primary elements. The herbs—more accurately "medicinals," as they often include minerals and animal parts—are almost always used in combination.

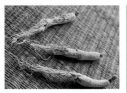

Ginseng
One of the most popular of all herbs, it is said to boost energy, ward off mental decline, and aid digestion.

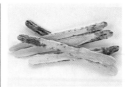

Astragalus Also known as yellow vetch, it purportedly bolsters the immune system. There are claims that it helps digestion and the lungs.

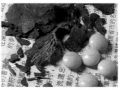

Fo Ti
A restorative said to strengthen the lower back, darken gray hair, and nourish semen and blood.

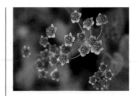

Buplerurum
Used for a variety of liver diseases, including cirrhosis and hepatitis.

NATIVE AMERICAN

To the early indigenous populations of North and South America, plants, stones, and animals provided as much healing information as any of today's medical tomes. Their herbal remedies tended to be antimicrobial.

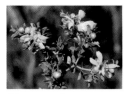

Chaparral Has been purported to offer anti-viral, antifungal, and antibacterial protections on top of an anti-inflammatory action. Warning: Can be dangerous if not prepared properly, causing serious liver damage.

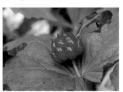

Goldenseal Used as an antibiotic and to clear the gastrointestinal tract of harmful yeast and bacteria. May have anti-mucus properties as well. Not safe for children or pregnant or lactating women.

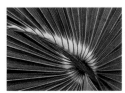

Saw palmetto Reputation for treating prostate problems, but studies yield conflicting results. Used also for impotence and upper respiratory problems.

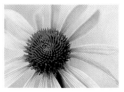

Echinacea Another antibiotic, said to activate white blood cells. A popular treatment for the common cold, though studies have generally failed to confirm its effectiveness.

EUROPEAN

Old World herbs have often served as a bridge between older, Eastern holistic traditions and the symptom-based approach of modern medicine. They are prescribed primarily as antidotes for the excesses of modern living.

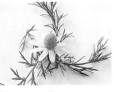

Chamomile Used to calm the nervous system and digestive tract.

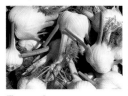

Fennel Said to relieve intestinal bloating and gas.

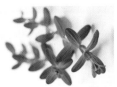

St. John's wort Has been shown to treat mild depression, but also interferes with some prescription drugs. Those taking medications should not begin to use it without consulting a doctor.

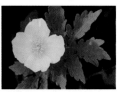

Celandine Used as an all-encompassing liver remedy, as well as a treatment for gout and insomnia.

COMMON GROUND

Several broad-based herbs span most traditions, though they often have different names in different cultures.

Ginger Digestive that dissolves mucus. Good results for motion sickness.

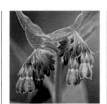

Comfrey Also called "knitbone," because of its reputation for healing fractures. For topical use only; can be toxic if taken internally.

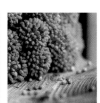

Angelica The Chinese variety (dong gui) is considered a first-line treatment for female disorders related to menstruation and pregnancy.

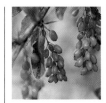

Barberry Said to dissolve kidney stones and clear gout.

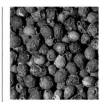

Hawthorn Berries Used to treat atherosclerotic heart disease. Considered a digestive by the Chinese.

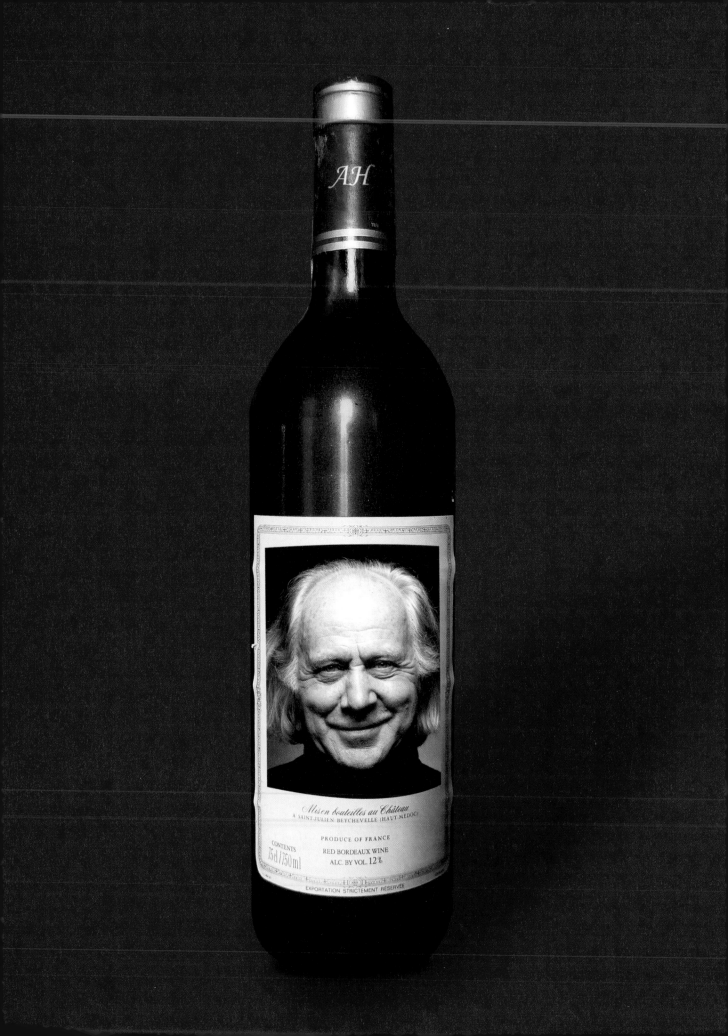

Aging Well

How to Keep Your Mind Sharp

As we age, our brains tend to decline in size and speed, but these seven healthy habits can make a real difference. **By Roseann Foley Henry**

UNCLE JAMES WAS ONE AMAZING GUY. CLOSE TO 80, HE COULD STILL recount events from decades ago with clarity and precision—and even humor. Nor did he miss a beat when conversation shifted from the good old days to current events, clearly articulating his position on the harmful effects of government subsidies on local farms. He lived by himself, shopped for himself, drove himself where he needed to go. Uncle James was ... sharp.

Of course, he wouldn't have been nearly so amazing if he'd been 40. We expect older folks to be a bit fuzzy, having lost some of their mental edge over the march of time. And many of us—as we help Dad download an app or show Mom how to use the remote—dread the prospect of losing it ourselves. We hope for continued physical health, yes, but what good will it do if we don't have our marbles? At the very least, we want to know we won't end up staring in befuddlement at whatever electronic gadget is the rage when we hit 75.

What we think of as sharpness—the cognitive ability to choose a health plan, use

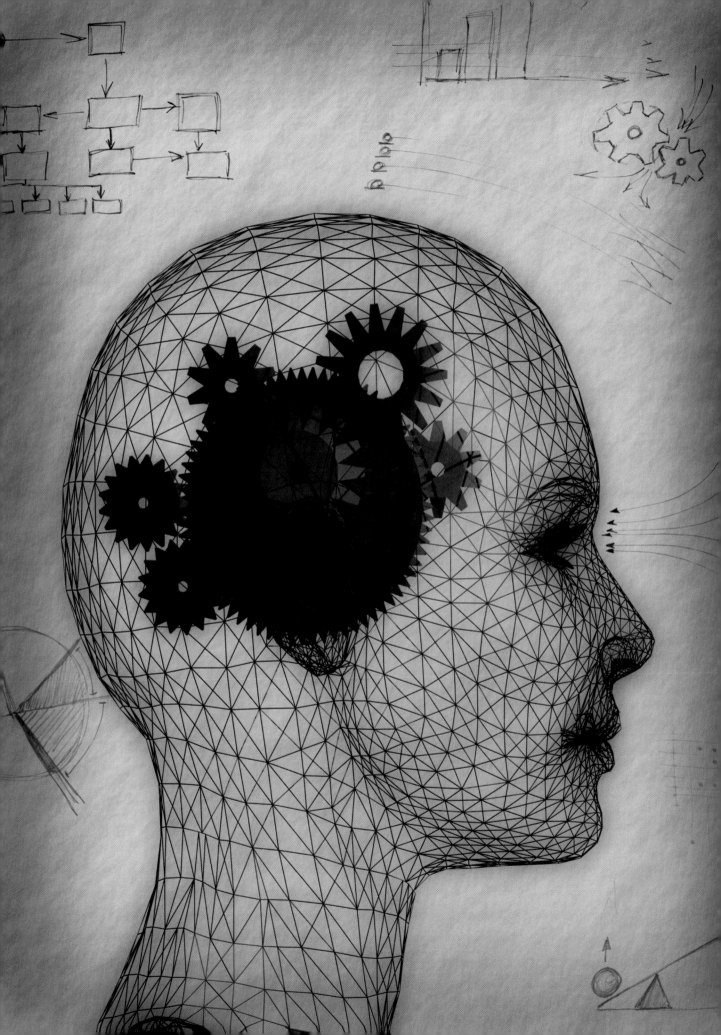

a new cellphone, or understand a joke—is regulated in the cerebral cortex, the deeply wrinkled layer of gray matter on the outside of the brain. And the older we get, the less cortex we have. A 2004 study found that the thickness, volume, and surface area of the cortex of healthy individuals go down with age. That shrinkage starts distressingly early too; 30-year-olds already show signs of thinning, and by 60 the reduction is pronounced.

That's not the only damage to worry about, either. An aging brain loses not only gray matter, but also some of the white matter below it. Myelin is the insulating fatty material that coats axons, the fibers that carry messages throughout the brain, and its scarcity is implicated in many neurodegenerative diseases, including Alzheimer's. But the loss of myelin also occurs in healthy but aging brains, and that loss is believed to slow processing speed and decrease the number of neural connections. That explains why the elderly, on average, do worse on tasks that require paying attention to lots of stimuli at the same time (like driving), holding multiple pieces of information simultaneously (like planning a trip to a new destination), and memory retrieval (like remembering where the car is parked at the mall).

Age-related changes to the brain's topography aren't the only threats. As the body goes, so goes the brain. Consider, for example, inflammation, our immune system's response to injury. Chronic inflammation takes a toll on aging bodies, causing cancer, heart disease, diabetes, and cognitive problems. Similarly, in the brain it has been linked broadly to conditions including depression, Alzheimer's, and Parkinson's.

Then again, as Uncle James and so many others like him prove, a free fall into feeblemindedness is not inevitable. "You can clearly see the loss of volume in older brains," says Philip Stieg, professor and chairman of the department of neurological surgery at Weill Cornell Medical College and neurosurgeon-in-chief at New York–Presbyterian Hospital. Stieg has seen more than his share of brains. "What you don't see is a strict correlation between that physical change and cognitive changes. You can have normal cognitive function even as the brain loses volume." So why do some seniors stay sharp, while others don't? Are their brains shrinking less, or are they doing something to compensate?

As it turns out, it's a bit of both. Recent stud-

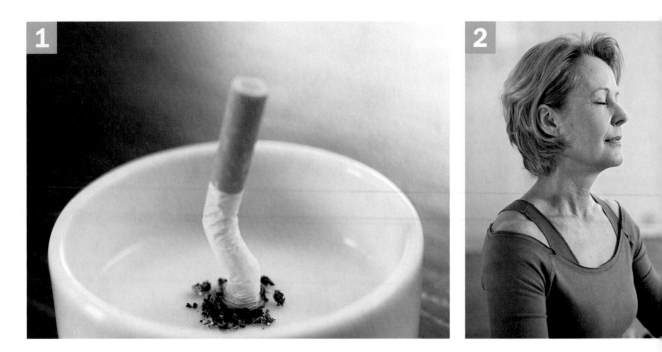

ies have shown that the adult brain is not, as had long been believed, unchangeable. Rather, it is neuroplastic—subject to physical modifications caused by life experiences and environmental factors. Scientists have also proved that the adult brain is capable of neurogenesis, the process of creating new cells, even as it loses volume. Finally, while brains often lose volume, speed, and efficiency as the years pass, there's a lot of variation in how much and how fast. Put it all together and it spells serious hope for aging brains.

With possibility, though, comes responsibility. Brains don't heal themselves. Industry has heeded the call, offering pharmaceuticals, supplements, even videogames, that promise to keep us savvy and sharp. But not even a magic pill can counteract the effects of age if the person taking it engages in a lifestyle that accelerates those effects.

The research is full of correlations (for instance, people with robust blood flow in the brain perform cognitive tasks better) but a locked-down cause and effect is rare (is it actually better flow that gives those people their better function?). Still, there are some pretty well-established con-

nections, and they can provide sound direction on the path to a sharper old age.

1 STOP SMOKING

Everyone knows smoking is terribly damaging to the body. Well, it's just as awful for the brain. A 2010 study showed that the cerebral cortex of smokers was significantly thinner than that of nonsmokers. Also, cortical thickness was directly correlated with the number of cigarettes and duration of the habit. Smoking effectively ages brains prematurely.

2 MANAGE STRESS

A little stress every now and then is inevitable, and in fact challenging situations can push brains to heightened competency. But chronic negative stress releases chemicals that inhibit neurogenesis and can cause adverse physical changes in the brain. Yoga is one potential antidote because it reduces levels of the stress hormone cortisol and acts as a natural anti-inflammatory. Meditation is another: Amit Sood, director of research and practice at the Mayo Clinic's Complementary and Integrative Medicine Program, uses meditation techniques to

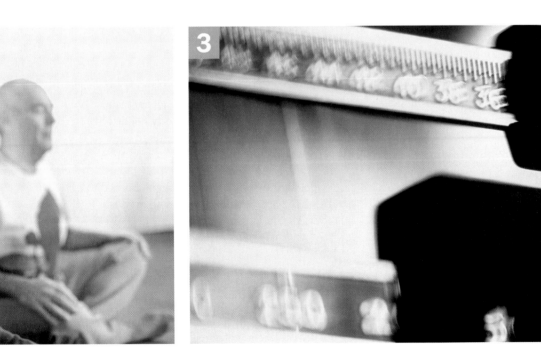

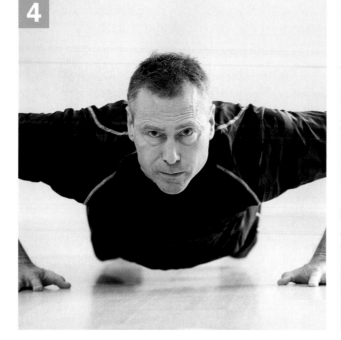

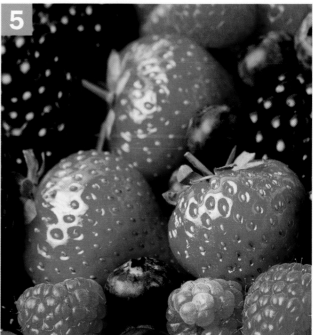

help patients better cope with adversity. "Anxiety and depression affect the limbic system, which governs emotion, behavior, and long-term memory," says Sood. "Meditation works by teaching patients to fully engage in the moment, which can calm the limbic system and increase activity in the higher cortical brain."

There are pictures to support that theory: A 2005 study showed that participants who meditated over a long period had thicker cortices than those who didn't. A more recent study found improvement in the white matter of subjects who had completed as little as four weeks of integrative body-mind training.

3 STAY TRIM

A higher body mass index has been linked to lower brain volume in the elderly. It's a sad fact: the bigger the waistline, the smaller the brain. Researchers don't know why—it could be that the same genetic variation leads to both obesity and atrophy, or it could be that a high-fat diet causes both. Couple this with the deleterious effects of obesity's companions, high blood pressure and diabetes, and going lean is an obvious choice.

4 KEEP MOVING

The brain isn't a muscle, but it can benefit from a workout. Exercise increases the flow of blood, and the oxygen and nutrients it carries, to the brain. Also, physical exertion causes the release of brain-derived neurotrophic factor, a protein that bolsters existing neurons and encourages the growth of new ones.

As Joy Bauer, a leading diet and fitness expert who is the nutrition and health editor for the *Today Show*, puts it, "A healthy heart is a healthy brain. Every cell in the body needs a steady supply of oxygen and nutrients to work properly, and a healthy heart keeps those supply lines open. Anything that impedes blood flow—like high blood pressure or high cholesterol—will have a terrible effect on all organs, including the brain."

5 EAT RIGHT

You can boost brainpower through diet too. In particular, emphasize choices that include antioxidants and inflammation fighters. Antioxidants capture free radicals, molecules that can set off a chain reaction of damage to a variety of

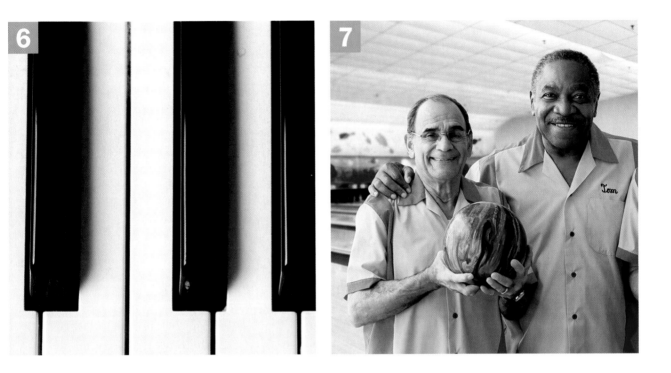

6

7

cells, and that includes brain cells. Dark-colored fruits and vegetables give you the biggest antioxidant bang for the buck. Likewise, seek out foods that counter inflammation, such as those rich in omega-3 fatty acids, like fish and plant oils. And avoid foods that trigger inflammatory responses, such as sugars, processed foods, alcohol, and refined grains.

If this prescription for brain wellness sounds familiar, that's because it is. The habits that will keep you sharp in your old age are just the ones that will help get you there in the first place. But there is more work to do. Minds can get lazy. So use your brain as much as possible. Do active cognitive tasks and maintain a vibrant social life. As we age, it's too easy to retire into solitude, just us and our TV. We need to get out there, to keep working our brains. And that leads to the two final pieces of advice:

6 KEEP LEARNING

Novel intellectual tasks, from puzzle solving to learning a new instrument or language, stimulate the brain to form new connections. Learning to juggle, for example, has been shown

to trigger at least short-term structural changes in the brain. Longer-term results are harder to pin down. Often, brain-training exercises primarily help people perform a particular task better. So doing the daily crossword will improve your crossword-solving skills, but don't count on it to help you program the TV remote.

7 STAY CONNECTED

Keeping up with friends, or making new ones, requires the brain to perform mental tasks such as recognizing faces, recalling names, following conversations, and producing appropriate responses. And that doesn't even include the emotional support that a network of friends can provide.

Which brings us back to Uncle James. He never set foot in a gym or played online brain games. But he did eat well and he always seemed calm. And until the day he died, he knew how to work a room, bantering with people half his age. To be sure, no one ever actually measured his cortex. But it was obvious to anyone paying attention that the man who never lost a debate definitely won his battle against aging.

Which Way To the Fountain Of Youth?

Scientists now know exactly what breaks down in our bodies and causes us to age. To find a way to slow this process, they're heading to far-flung destinations to uncover the secrets of their long-lived residents. *By M.A. Landau*

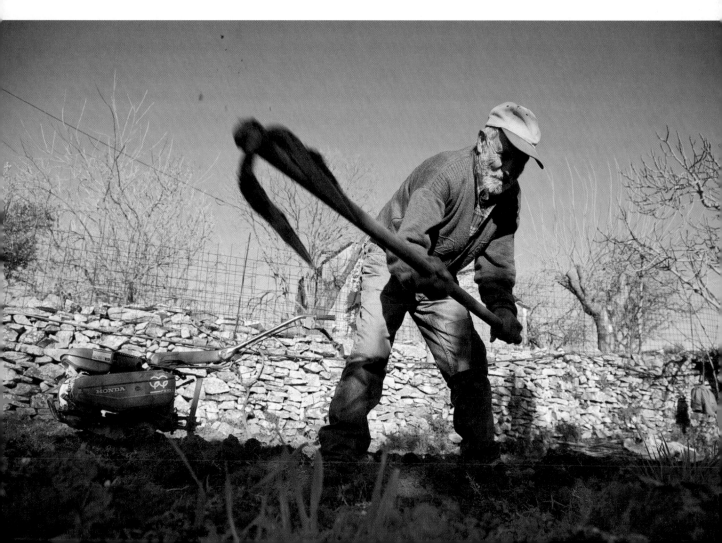

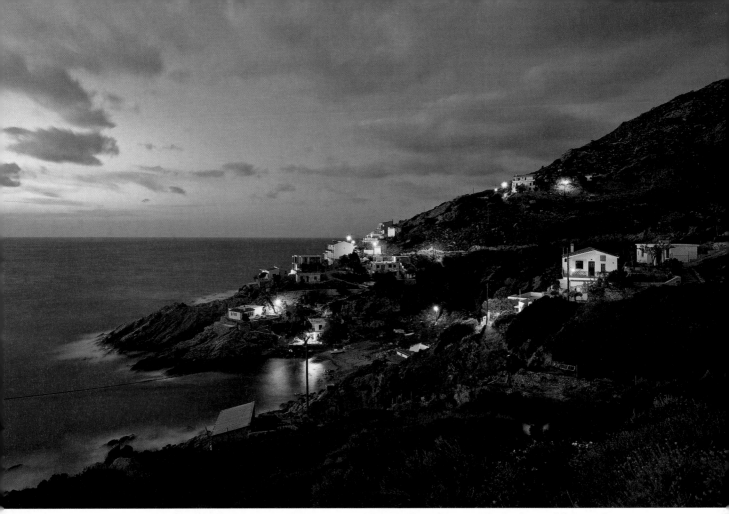

Above: Residents of places like Okinawa, Japan; Nicoya, Costa Rica; and Ikaria, Greece (above and throughout), celebrate 100th birthdays 10 times more often than people in the rest of the world. Below left: This Greek nonagenerian, who gave his name only as Jorgos, keeps up a weekly routine of tilling his land.

I F ONLY THERE WERE A WAY TO BE YOUNG AGAIN. WHO KNOWS WHO HAD THAT thought first, but it had to have been one of our earliest ancestors, right? Some sluggish adult cave dweller as he jealously watched his exuberant offspring fresh from a hunt. It's a wish that has grown no less poignant over the millennia. It has, however, most assuredly grown more prevalent, now that 81 million baby boomers are poised to cross the threshold into their senior years, with another 61 million Gen Xers right behind.

Despite intensive investigation, though, no pill or potion has yet proved that it can turn back the clock of our complex physiology. Of course, you wouldn't know it from all the hype that routinely accompanies whatever hormone or superberry is the ingestible du jour. The Internet has especially become fertile ground for the empty promises of all the anti-aging-therapy-mongers. There really does seem to be enough quackery being peddled these days to transform every fading middle-ager into a strong and sexy 20-year-old—better, even, than he was the first time around. But evidence to support the various claims is thin at best, often based on a positive effect on the lifespan or general well-being of fruit flies or lab rodents. The safety data are thinner still. Even if future studies vindicate some of these therapies, their specific effects—boosting libido, for example—will probably keep them a mere footnote in the quest for a longer, healthier life. Fortunately, more mainstream science is helping to draw a different map to the fountain of youth.

We typically date ourselves by the lines on our face, the aches in our knees, or the strength of our bifocals. But researchers have uncovered a more accurate measure. Hidden deep inside the body's cells, they're called telomeres, and they are so important to every cell's aging process that the team that discovered their existence was awarded the Nobel Prize in medicine in 2009. Telomeres are sequences of DNA at the ends of each chromosome; they shorten over time—whenever a cell divides—until they cease to be. And when they no longer exist, the cell dies.

However, an enzyme called telomerase can restore some length to the chromosome, thus prolonging cell life. And that bit of information has spurred a hunt for interventions that may increase the production of telomerase. The secret to such interventions, it seems, winds through the fabric of our day-to-day experiences—urging us to examine, and in many cases, transform, the way we live.

As it turns out, unhealthy habits—smoking,

Reaping what they sow: Eleftheria, shown here at 92, and her centenarian husband grow herbs in their garden. Close family relationships, productive work, and healthy eating habits have been shown to increase longevity.

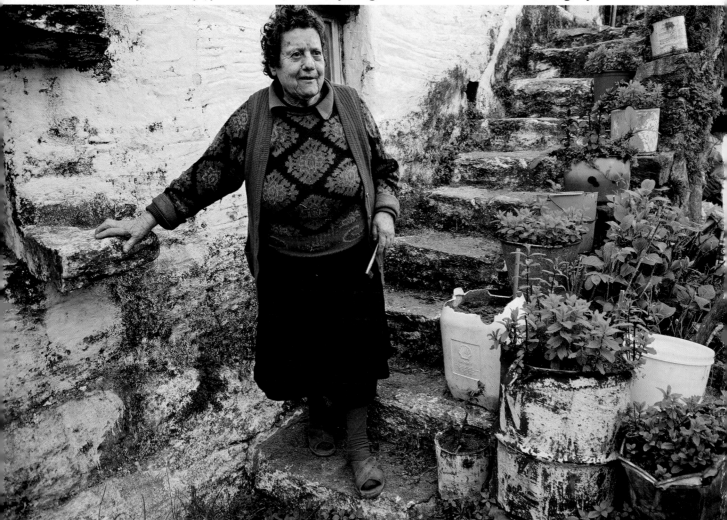

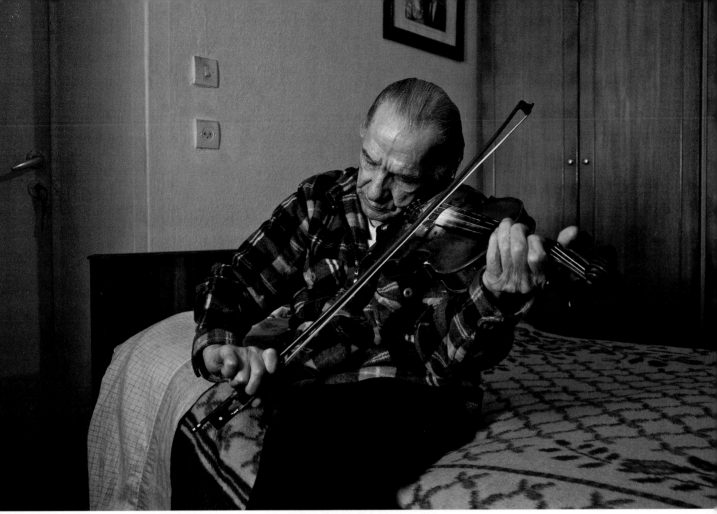

Living with a purpose: Yoannis has played the violin all his long life, and while his sight is almost gone, his hearing has stayed sharp—and so has he.

overeating, and the like—have been linked to premature telomere shortening. And at least one intriguing study suggests that a comprehensive lifestyle approach, one that features behaviors long known to promote general wellness, could be just what the doctor ordered. A mere three months after overhauling their daily regimens, study participants had significant increases in telomerase activity, an impressive 30%.

Although the research, by Dean Ornish and fellow scientists at the University of California at San Francisco, involved only men with early prostate cancer, the results offer tantalizing possibilities for all of us. The participants made considerable changes to their routines: They followed a very low-fat diet full of vegetables, fruits, beans, and whole grains; they exercised moderately for 30 minutes on most days; they attended a weekly communal support group; and they reduced stress through a daily hourlong program of yoga, guided imagery, meditation, and other relaxation techniques. While it is impossible to tease out which of those components had the

greatest effects, all of them probably played a role, says study co-author Jennifer Daubenmier. In any case, the research points to previously hidden biological processes, and the results seem to confirm that how we live has much to do with how long we live.

Support for this multipronged lifestyle approach is emerging as well from studies of the world's oldest old. Residents of places like Okinawa, Japan; Ikaria, Greece; and Nicoya, Costa Rica, celebrate their 100th birthday some 10 times more often than the worldwide average. Good genes, it turns out, account for only a fraction of that longevity. Despite vast differences in those far-flung, tradition-laden cultures, residents have surprisingly similar habits, says Dan Buettner, who chronicled those similarities in his book, *The Blue Zones: Lessons for Living Longer from the People Who've Lived the Longest*. While this type of observational research doesn't exactly provide the impeccable evidence of a clinical trial, Buettner's insights do offer a plausible strategy for living longer. Among his findings:

Long-lived people eat low and slow. Like the eating plan in the San Francisco study, diets in these cultures revolve around plant-based foods, especially vegetables, whole grains, and beans. (They do eat meat, but not too much and mostly on special occasions.) The islanders keep portion size reasonable too. Okinawan elders, for example, are quick to offer this advice: "*Hara hachi bu,*" or "Eat until you are 80% full."

They don't sit still. Moderate, sustained movement is inevitable when you spend your days toiling in the fields or among your herds.

Buettner suggests that Westerners mimic this kind of activity by planting a vegetable garden, taking walks at lunchtime, and putting away step-saving gadgets like the TV remote, garage door opener, and power mower.

They search for meaning. Lifelong commitments to family, community, and faith provide a natural buffer in these cultures against harmful life-shortening stressors. A sense of purpose keeps them young too. It's what the Nicoyans call *plan de vida*, or roughly, "why I wake up in the morning." So, too, does the savoring of

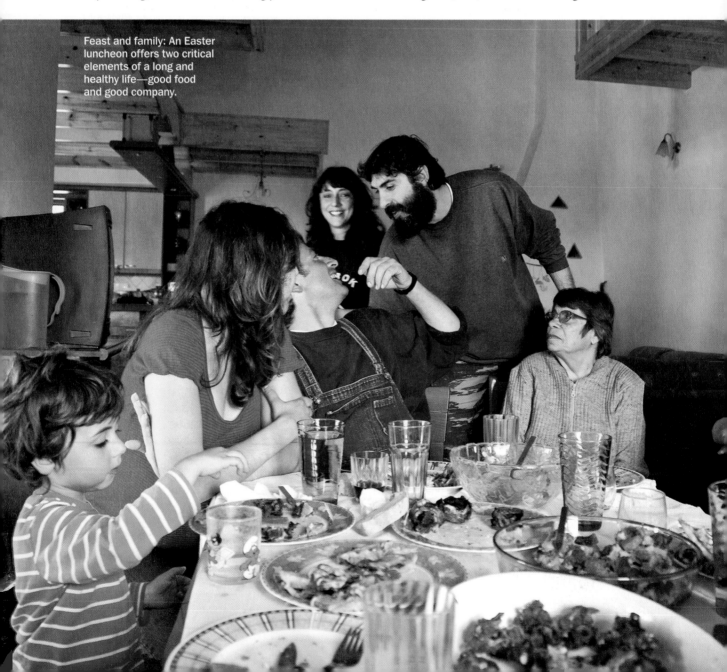

Feast and family: An Easter luncheon offers two critical elements of a long and healthy life—good food and good company.

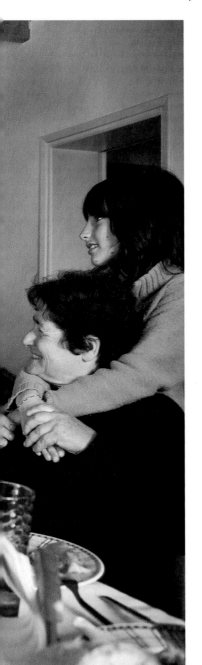

small joys: Witness the elderly shepherd who still pauses to appreciate the same sweeping vista he has gazed upon for most of his 80 years.

When you get right down to it, what's the point of living longer if all it adds up to is a few more years of frailty? That's why scientists at Mayo Clinic and elsewhere are also turning their sights on something they've dubbed "healthspan," the part of life you spend being vital and active.

This line of research is in its infancy, but it has already isolated key threats to healthspan. According to Nathan LeBrasseur, a rehabilitation specialist at Mayo, those include physical and mental disability, chronic disease, and the inability to bounce back from illness or injury. And one intervention didn't take long to prove its worth. It just happens to be one that influences lifespan as well: exercise. Physical activity pumps up muscle quantity, which matters because beginning in our forties we start to lose what eventually will be an average of 30% of muscle mass.

A growing body of research suggests that exercise also affects muscle quality by limiting the creation of damaging fatty deposits, which can infiltrate a muscle's fibers. Although getting on the workout bandwagon early is probably the single best way to promote healthspan, says LeBrasseur, "the good news is, it is never too late." Results from a small study by the National Institute on Aging, for one, suggest that gains can come even from training that starts when a person is in his eighties.

There you have it—the most important part of any trip to the fountain of youth is the hike you have to take to get there.

Forever Young

Drink this. Don't eat that. Take a couple of these. Lots of people have lots of theories about how you can slow the ravages of time. So far, though, many purported youth potions have proved less than miraculous. A capsule review:

Resveratrol. This compound, found in tiny amounts in red grapes and wine, captured the public imagination a couple of years back when overweight mice seemed to thrive on it. But subsequent findings contradict resveratrol's ability to prolong life. Says James Kirkland, a professor of aging research at Mayo Clinic: "Despite being studied intensively, there is no evidence that it affects lifespan."

Dehydroepiandrosterone (DHEA). The level of this hormone, which the body converts to estrogen and testosterone, starts to decline when we hit our twenties. But little evidence supports the notion that replenishing our stores with supplements slows aging. Plus, if you take too much, you risk hair loss, hypertension, and maybe even liver disease.

Human growth hormone (HGH) and testosterone. Prescribing these two hormones, which we produce less of as we age, is big business at anti-aging clinics. Some patients report feeling more youthful after taking them, and at least one small study found that testosterone enhanced mood, energy, and libido. But the risks of taking them long term are unknown, and might even include consequences as serious as cancer.

Acetyl-L-carnitine (ALCAR). Derived from an amino acid, this compound has been found in rats to reverse decay in mitochondria, the energy producers in every cell. In one small study in older men, ALCAR supplementation helped fight fatigue and sexual decline. While it appears to be safe, larger studies may tell whether daily doses for general health can be recommended.

Calorie restriction. "Of all the anti-aging strategies, this has the most evidence going for it," says Brent Bauer, director of the Mayo Clinic Integrative Medicine Program. Dramatically cutting calories by up to 40% of daily requirements has lengthened the lives of yeast, fruit flies, mice, and rats. In one human study, 48 calorie-slashers (who did get all the necessary nutrients) improved two markers associated with longevity: lower fasting insulin levels and body temperature. Will those subjects actually live longer? We'll have to wait and see. But even if they do, will the price—constant low-grade hunger—be too high for most of us?

A History Of Hooey

Scientific nonsense has often spurred legitimate medical progress. But it's not always easy to tell the difference between the two.
By Jeffrey Kluger and David Bjerklie

I F YOU'RE A GUY SUFFERING FROM ERECTILE DYSFUNCTION, HERE'S A PIECE OF advice you can take to the bank: Stay away from goat testicles. And if that seems self-evident to you—and not just because the goats might have something to say about it—be assured that such common sense was not always the case.

In the 1920s, John Foster Brinkley, a North Carolina physician who had been a Confederate army medic in the Civil War, grew wealthy hawking patent medicine, hosting a radio show, and, yes, transplanting goat testicles into patients who were having trouble maintaining their "manly vigor." Not surprisingly, the treatments produced—how best to put this?—imperfect results, leading to serious infections and even death. Not surprisingly either, the good doctor wound up discredited and penniless—but not before starting an amateur baseball team he called the Brinkley Goats, proving that even in the 1920s disgraced people weren't big on shame.

Brinkley might have been one of history's most obvious quacks, but quackery has always been around. It was in 1895 that Norwegian surgeon Alex Cappelin first cracked open a chest and operated on a beating heart. He seems like a hero now, but how would you have liked to be the first patient on his table? The difference between a Cappelin and a Brinkley is not the outrageous-ness of their ideas but the fact that one of them turned out to be grounded in science while the other was full of reckless nonsense.

Yet even in nonsense there can be grains of wisdom. Brinkley was a charlatan, but looking for ways to use tissue from animals to help treat human beings is a robust area of modern medical research, though today we give it a niftier name—xenotransplantation—and we don't dare let any of it go mainstream until we've worked out all the infection and rejection issues first.

We're seeing something similar—though in a far more benign way—with alternative and complementary medicine. The ancient healer who drove out disease by chanting may make you roll your eyes, but from that original practice flowed the idea of music therapy—which science has shown does work. The mystical laying-on of hands may not have a long history of success, but therapeutic massage does. The history of medicine is a long march of brilliant ideas, terrible ideas, and some that have turned out to be both. Here are a few of the high—and low—moments. Mental illness has never been an easy problem to treat, but a few millennia ago, doctors believed they had just the thing: trepanning. The thinking—such as it was—behind this practice was that because madness was surely caused by evil spirits, and the only sensible place for them to live was in the head, all you had to do was drill a few holes in the skull and let them out. Hard to argue with that—and apparently few people did. Archeological evidence suggests that trepanning had a run of some 10,000 years—grim years, no doubt, for the patients. Yet what the ancients learned from that dubious practice gave them some of humanity's first insights into the anatomy of the cranium and helped lead to the modern practice of temporarily removing portions of the skull to accommodate swelling and prevent permanent damage after brain injury.

Bloodletting was another common—and messy—treatment. Created by both the ancient Egyptians and the Greeks, the practice was based on the belief that an imbalance of the body's four humors—black bile, yellow bile, phlegm, and blood—was the cause of all illness and that draining some of the blood would bring things back in line. That, alas, turned out not to be so, as the countless people killed over the centuries by the practice proved. The unhappy list of victims includes George Washington, who may have had more than half of his blood drained during the treatment of what was—no coincidence here—his final illness. The regrettable track record of bloodletting notwithstanding, 21st-century doctors now know that periodic and controlled bleeding can in fact be helpful in treating hemochromatosis (abnormal iron accumulation) and polycythemia vera (an overproduction of red blood cells). Science's modern understanding of the brain has its roots in long-ago medical hogwash as

well. In the 18th century German physician Franz Anton Mesmer argued that a natural energy pervades all things—a life-giving charge he called "animal magnetism," which powers the body like electricity. His theory hung around for 200 years, and by the early 20th century Mesmer-inspired electric coils were in wide circulation to treat, well, whatever the huckster selling the things said they did.

Such useless gadgetry fell out of favor, but electricity and magnetism have shown some medical potential. Severe depression can be successfully treated by electroconvulsive therapy (particularly the newer iterations that dispense with a lot of the "convulsive" part), as well as by transcranial magnetic stimulation, a relatively new, noninvasive way to repolarize neurons in the brain and, in some cases, improve mood. The very idea that electricity drives the body is at the root of our modern grasp of how the nervous system operates, and has led to the development of a new generation of functional prostheses.

In fairness to scientists blinkered by their times, it's often impossible to recognize a deeply bad idea until you've acted on it and seen the damage it can do. And it can be easy to err too far in the other direction, concluding that the risks of medical progress outweigh the rewards. In 1891, physician and professor Oliver Wendell Holmes, disturbed by toxins such as mercury and strychnine that were being used in medicines, famously wrote, "I firmly believe that ... if the whole *materia medica*, as now used, could be sunk to the bottom of the sea, it would be all the better for mankind—and all the worse for the fishes."

Clearly, that would have been a bad move. If the long arc of medical science has taught us anything, it's that healing—for all its fitful progress—can come from the most improbable places. True wisdom means keeping a mind that's both open and skeptical, empirical and intuitive—admitting that we can never be entirely sure what it will take to make us well, but resolving to take advantage of it when we see it.

About the Authors

LESLEY ALDERMAN is a health writer and certified yoga instructor. She was a health editor at *Real Simple* and co-wrote the Patient Money column for the *New York Times*. Her first book, *The Book of Times*, will be published in January by HarperCollins.

BRENT BAUER is the director of the Mayo Clinic Integrative Medicine Program and the medical editor of the *Mayo Clinic Book of Alternative Medicine*.

DAVID BJERKLIE has been a senior reporter at TIME, a senior editor at *Time for Kids*, and a science writer/editor at TheVisualMD.com. He is also the author of children's books on butterflies, agriculture, and environmental justice.

JOHN CLOUD is a staff writer for TIME and has written dozens of in-depth features, including cover pieces on organic food, gay teenagers, and such diverse figures as Ann Coulter and Howard Dean.

STACEY COLINO writes about health and psychological issues for *Real Simple, More, Parents,* and other magazines. Her most recent book is *Eat! Move! Play! A Parent's Guide for Raising Healthy, Happy Kids*.

ELIZABETH DIAS is a writer-reporter in TIME's Washington bureau and covers religion and politics.

ROSEANN FOLEY HENRY is a freelance writer and editor who specializes in health and wellness. Her work has appeared in *Discover*, PsychologyToday.com, and many other publications.

BETH HOWARD writes about health, medicine, and wellness for many national publications, including *US News & World Report, AARP: The Magazine, Reader's Digest,* and *Prevention*.

JEFFREY KLUGER is a senior editor who oversees TIME's science, health, and technology reporting. He has written or co-written nearly 40 cover stories for the magazine and regularly contributes articles and commentary on science and health stories.

M.A. LANDAU writes about alternative medicine for many national magazines.

LORI OLIWENSTEIN is a freelance science writer and editor living in Los Angeles. She is the author of *Taming Bipolar Disorder* (2004).

ALICE PARK is a staff writer at TIME. Since 1993 she has reported on the frontiers of health and medicine in articles covering issues such as AIDS, cancer, and Alzheimer's.

PEG ROSEN writes frequently about health and fitness for websites and national magazines. She blogs at www.relish-this.blogspot.com.

BRYAN WALSH is a senior editor for TIME INTERNATIONAL. He also writes the Going Green column for TIME and Time.com and contributes to Time.com's environmental issues blog, Ecocentric.

Credits